CHAIR YOGA REVOLUTION

A Comprehensive Guide for Seniors
to Enhance Mobility, Strength, and Independence

Alexandra Grace

FOR THE FIRST 100 ONLY

CLAIM

YOUR BONUS

NOW

Table of Contents

Chapter 1:

Introduction to Yoga Chair

Embracing the Golden Years with Grace and Strength

Welcome to "Chair Yoga Revolution," a beacon of light for seniors seeking to reclaim their autonomy, enhance their physical capabilities, and enrich their golden years with joy and vitality. This guide is not merely a collection of exercises; it is a journey towards a more fulfilling, active, and independent life.

In the twilight years of life, it's easy to succumb to the narrative that aging equates to decline – a loss of mobility, strength, and independence. However, this book stands as a testament to the contrary, illuminating a path of empowerment through the gentle, yet profoundly effective practice of chair yoga.

Why Chair Yoga?

Chair yoga emerges as a revolutionary approach, meticulously adapted to meet the unique needs of seniors. It bridges the gap between the desire for physical activity and the challenges that come with age. With a chair as your steadfast companion, this practice offers a safe, accessible, and versatile method to enhance your well-being, irrespective of your current fitness level or mobility constraints.

The Power of Adaptability

Chair yoga's beauty lies in its adaptability. Each pose, stretch, and breathing technique has been tailored to provide maximum benefits without the risk of injury. This guide demystifies yoga, transforming it from an intimidating art form into a welcoming, inclusive practice that you can make a part of your daily routine.

A Holistic Approach to Well-being

"A Comprehensive Guide for Seniors to Enhance Mobility, Strength, and Independence" transcends physical exercise. It advocates for a holistic view of health, incorporating mindfulness, meditation, and nutritional advice to nourish both the body and soul. This holistic approach ensures a balanced path to wellness, catering not just to physical health but to mental and emotional well-being as well.

Your Journey Begins

This book is your guide through the transformative practice of chair yoga. It will lead you through the fundamentals, from setting up your practice space to mastering each pose with confidence. It celebrates your progress, encouraging you to embrace each movement as a step towards greater mobility, strength, and independence.

A Testament to Resilience and Joy

This book is more than a manual; it's a celebration of life's resilience and the joy of movement. It's a reminder that age is but a number, and with each breath and stretch, you're capable of rediscovering the vitality within.

Join the Revolution

The chair yoga revolution is about breaking barriers, challenging stereotypes about aging, and redefining what it means to grow older. It's about choosing to live your senior years with strength, grace, and independence. This book is your first step on a journey that promises transformation, empowerment, and a renewed zest for life.

Given the detailed outline provided earlier, let's further delve into the narrative for "Chair Yoga Revolution," expanding upon the themes introduced.

The Age of Empowerment

Aging is an inevitable part of life, a phase that's often accompanied by mixed feelings. While it brings wisdom and experiences, it can also introduce challenges to our physical health and mobility. However, the golden years are not a time to retreat but to embrace life with open arms. Chair yoga presents a beautiful opportunity to do just that, offering a gentle yet effective way to maintain and even enhance your physical and mental well-being.

The exercises and practices outlined in this book have been carefully selected and adapted to meet you where you are. Whether you're someone who's been active all your life or you're just beginning to incorporate physical activity into your daily routine, chair yoga is for you. It's a testament to the fact that it's never too late to start, and that every small step counts.

The Science of Well-being

Numerous studies have highlighted the benefits of regular physical activity for seniors, including improved mobility, balance, and overall quality of life. Chair yoga, with its focus on gentle stretching, strengthening, and balancing exercises, directly contributes to these outcomes. Furthermore, its emphasis on mindful breathing and meditation addresses the mental and emotional aspects of aging, helping to reduce stress, anxiety, and feelings of loneliness.

In this book, we delve into the science behind each pose and practice, explaining how they contribute to your health and why they're particularly beneficial as we age. This evidence-based approach ensures that you're not just following along but understanding the rationale behind each movement, making your practice even more meaningful.

Setting the Stage for Success

Before diving into the exercises, we'll guide you through setting up your practice space. Creating a safe, comfortable, and inviting environment is crucial to your success. We'll explore how to choose the right chair, how to position yourself for maximum benefit, and how to create a routine that fits seamlessly into your life.

This book is structured to gradually build your confidence and skills. Starting with basic poses and breathing exercises, we'll progressively move to more advanced practices. Each chapter builds upon the last, ensuring a natural progression that respects your body's pace and abilities.

A Community of Support

One of the most powerful aspects of embarking on this chair yoga journey is the sense of community it fosters. Though you may be practicing alone, you're joining a global movement of seniors choosing to live their best lives through yoga. This book serves as a bridge, connecting you to others who, just like you, are discovering the joy and freedom that comes with improved mobility and strength.

We encourage you to share your journey, challenges, and victories with friends, family, or fellow practitioners. The stories featured in this book—from people who have transformed their lives through chair yoga—serve as a reminder that you're not alone. Your progress, no matter how small it might seem, is a cause for celebration.

Your Path to Renewal

"Chair Yoga Revolution" is more than just a manual; it's a call to action. It's an invitation to view aging not as a decline but as a chapter rich with potential for growth, learning, and happiness. Through the practice of chair yoga, you're not just improving your physical health; you're embracing a holistic approach to well-being that nurtures your mind, body, and spirit.

As you turn each page and try each pose, remember that this book is a starting point. The true journey unfolds in daily practice, in the quiet moments of connection between your breath and movement, and in the joy of discovering what you're capable of.

Welcome to the Chair Yoga Revolution. Your adventure towards a more empowered, balanced, and fulfilling life begins now.

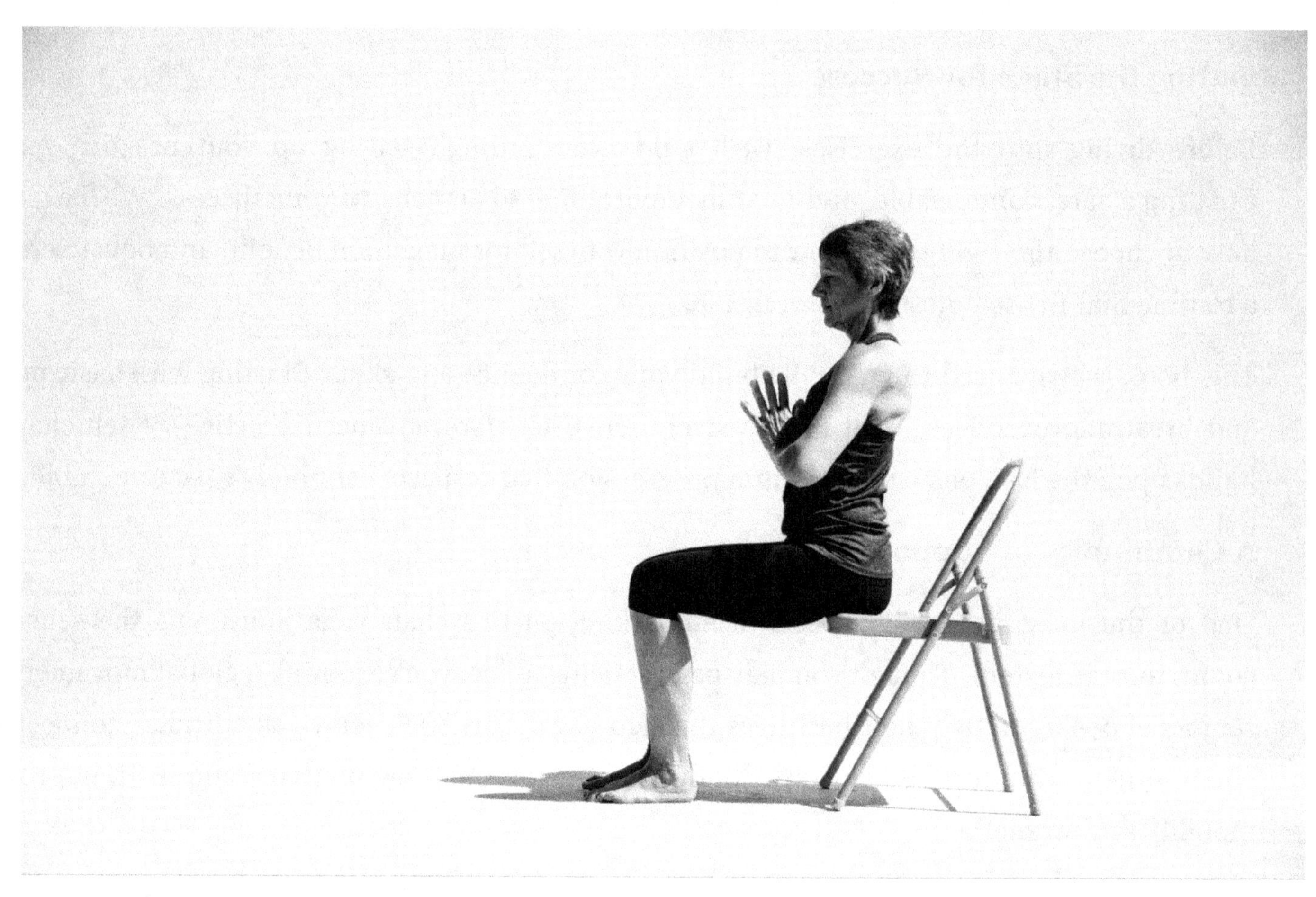

What is Chair Yoga? Understanding the Basics

Chair yoga is an innovative adaptation of traditional yoga that makes the extensive benefits of yoga accessible to a broader audience, especially seniors and individuals with mobility challenges. At its core, chair yoga embodies the essence of adaptability and inclusivity, providing a safe, gentle, and effective way to improve physical health, enhance mental clarity, and foster emotional well-being.

The Foundation of Chair Yoga

Chair yoga is built on the foundation of traditional yoga principles, which aim to unite the body, mind, and spirit through a combination of postures, breathing techniques, and meditation. However, chair yoga modifies these practices to be performed while seated in a chair or using a chair for support. This modification ensures that individuals who may have difficulty standing for extended periods or getting down on the floor can still enjoy the holistic benefits of yoga.

Key Components of Chair Yoga

1. Seated Poses: These form the backbone of chair yoga, allowing practitioners to perform a variety of stretches and movements without leaving their chairs. These poses target various body parts, including the neck, shoulders, arms, back, hips, and legs, promoting flexibility, strength, and circulation.
2. Standing and Supported Poses: For those who can stand, chair yoga incorporates poses that use the chair as a prop for balance and support. These poses help build strength in the legs and core, improve balance, and enhance mobility.

3. Breathing Exercises: Proper breathing is a critical element of chair yoga, as it is in all forms of yoga. Breathing exercises, or pranayama, are practiced to calm the mind, reduce stress, and improve lung function.
4. Mindfulness and Meditation: Chair yoga sessions often conclude with a period of relaxation and meditation, emphasizing mindfulness and promoting mental and emotional peace.

Benefits of Chair Yoga

The versatility of chair yoga makes it an effective form of exercise for improving overall health. Its benefits include:

Enhanced Flexibility: Regular practice helps increase range of motion, reducing stiffness and making daily activities easier.

Increased Strength: Poses designed to work various muscle groups build strength, which is crucial for maintaining independence.

Improved Balance and Stability: Balancing exercises strengthen the muscles that support the joints, reducing the risk of falls.

Stress Reduction: The meditative aspects of chair yoga help alleviate stress and anxiety, promoting a sense of calm.

Better Circulation: Gentle movements encourage blood flow, benefiting heart health and reducing swelling in the extremities.

Pain Relief: Many practitioners find relief from chronic pain conditions, such as arthritis, through regular chair yoga practice.

Getting Started with Chair Yoga

Embarking on a chair yoga journey requires little in the way of equipment—a sturdy, armless chair and comfortable clothing are all you need to begin. It is a practice that can be adapted to fit any fitness level, making it an excellent option for seniors looking to start exercising or anyone seeking a gentle form of physical activity.

Chair Yoga: A Path to Empowerment

Chair yoga offers more than just physical benefits; it is a path to empowerment, enabling practitioners to take control of their health and well-being. By making yoga accessible, chair yoga opens up a world of possibilities for improved quality of life, regardless of age or mobility level.

Conclusion

Understanding the basics of chair yoga is the first step toward embracing a practice that promises enhanced mobility, strength, and independence. It is a testament to the adaptability of yoga and its capacity to meet us exactly where we are in our fitness journey. Chair yoga is not just about adapting yoga poses to a chair; it's about adapting to the evolving needs of our bodies and minds as we age, ensuring that we can all enjoy the profound benefits of yoga throughout our lives.

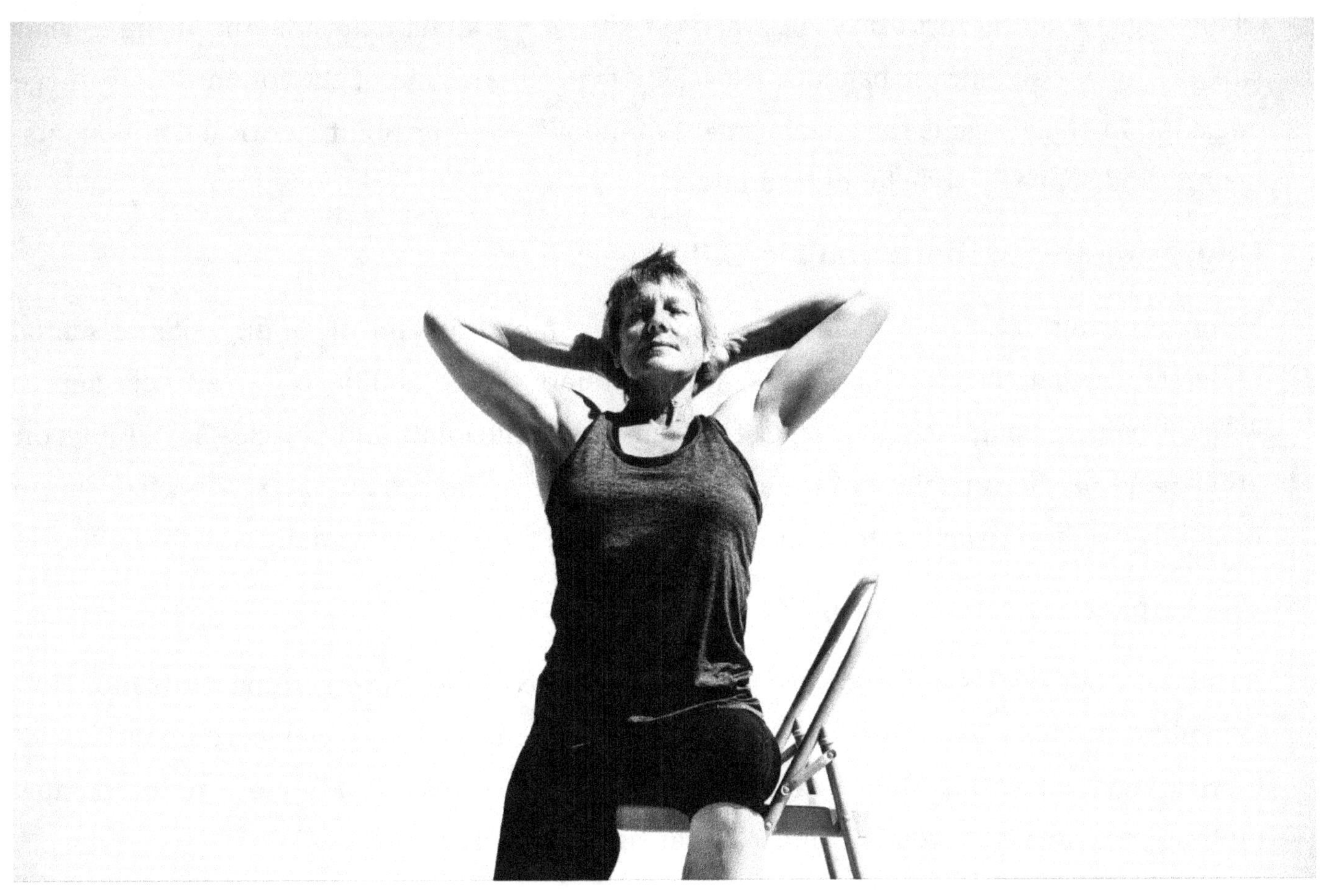

Chapter 2:

The Benefits of Chair Yoga for Seniors

Chair yoga offers a multitude of benefits tailored to meet the needs of seniors, making it an invaluable practice for enhancing overall well-being. By adapting traditional yoga poses for seated or supported standing positions, chair yoga makes the holistic advantages of yoga accessible to all. This chapter delves into the core benefits of chair yoga for seniors, highlighting how it enhances mobility and flexibility, builds strength and balance, reduces stress, improves mental health, promotes independence, and elevates the quality of life.

Enhancing Mobility and Flexibility

Chair yoga, a gentle form of yoga practiced sitting on a chair or standing using a chair for support, offers significant benefits, especially for seniors. One of the foremost advantages of engaging in chair yoga is the enhancement of mobility and flexibility, critical components of a healthy and active lifestyle for older adults.

Understanding Mobility and Flexibility

Before delving into how chair yoga enhances mobility and flexibility, it's essential to understand what these terms mean. Mobility refers to the ability to move freely and easily without pain, encompassing a range of movements in the joints and muscles. Flexibility, on the other hand, is the capability of the muscles to stretch. The two are interconnected; improved flexibility can lead to better mobility, which is crucial for performing daily activities effortlessly.

The Impact of Aging on Mobility and Flexibility

As we age, our bodies undergo various changes that can significantly impact our mobility and flexibility. Muscles tend to lose their mass and elasticity, joints can become stiff, and the lubricating fluid within them may decrease. These changes can lead to a reduced range of motion, pain during movement, and a higher risk of falls and injuries.

How Chair Yoga Comes into Play

Chair yoga offers a safe, accessible, and effective way to combat the limitations imposed by aging. By focusing on gentle stretching and strengthening exercises that can be done while seated or standing with the support of a chair, it targets key areas that contribute to mobility and flexibility.

Gentle Stretching

Chair yoga incorporates a variety of stretching exercises that target the major muscle groups. These stretches are designed to be gentle on the body, reducing the risk of overstretching or injury. By regularly engaging in these stretching exercises, seniors can gradually increase the length and elasticity of their muscles, which contributes to an enhanced range of motion in the joints.

For example, a simple seated forward bend can help stretch the spine, shoulders, and hamstrings, promoting flexibility in these areas. Similarly, a seated twist can improve the flexibility of the spine and shoulders, aiding in better rotation and side-to-side movement.

Strengthening Exercises

In addition to stretching, chair yoga includes exercises that strengthen the muscles surrounding the joints. Stronger muscles can better support the joints, leading to improved mobility. These exercises are tailored to be low-impact, focusing on building strength gradually without putting undue stress on the body.

For instance, leg lifts performed while seated can strengthen the thigh muscles and improve the flexibility and mobility of the hip joints. Arm raises can enhance shoulder mobility and flexibility, important for tasks that involve reaching or lifting.

Breathing Techniques and Mindfulness

Chair yoga also emphasizes the importance of breathing techniques and mindfulness in enhancing mobility and flexibility. Proper breathing can help to relax the muscles, making it easier to move into and hold stretches. Mindfulness, on the other hand, encourages an awareness of the body's limits, preventing overexertion and promoting a gentle approach to stretching and strengthening.

The Cumulative Benefits

The cumulative effect of regularly practicing chair yoga can be profound. Seniors can experience an improvement in their overall mobility, finding it easier to perform daily activities such as walking, bending, and reaching. Flexibility gains can lead to a decreased risk of muscle strains and joint pain, contributing to a higher quality of life.

Moreover, the enhanced mobility and flexibility fostered by chair yoga can contribute to better balance and a reduced risk of falls, a common concern among older adults. With increased confidence in their physical abilities, seniors can maintain their independence and continue to engage in activities they enjoy, promoting their physical and mental well-being.

In conclusion, chair yoga stands out as an accessible and effective way for seniors to enhance their mobility and flexibility. Through gentle stretching, strengthening exercises, and a focus on mindful breathing, chair yoga can help older adults overcome the limitations imposed by aging, leading to a more active, independent, and fulfilling life.

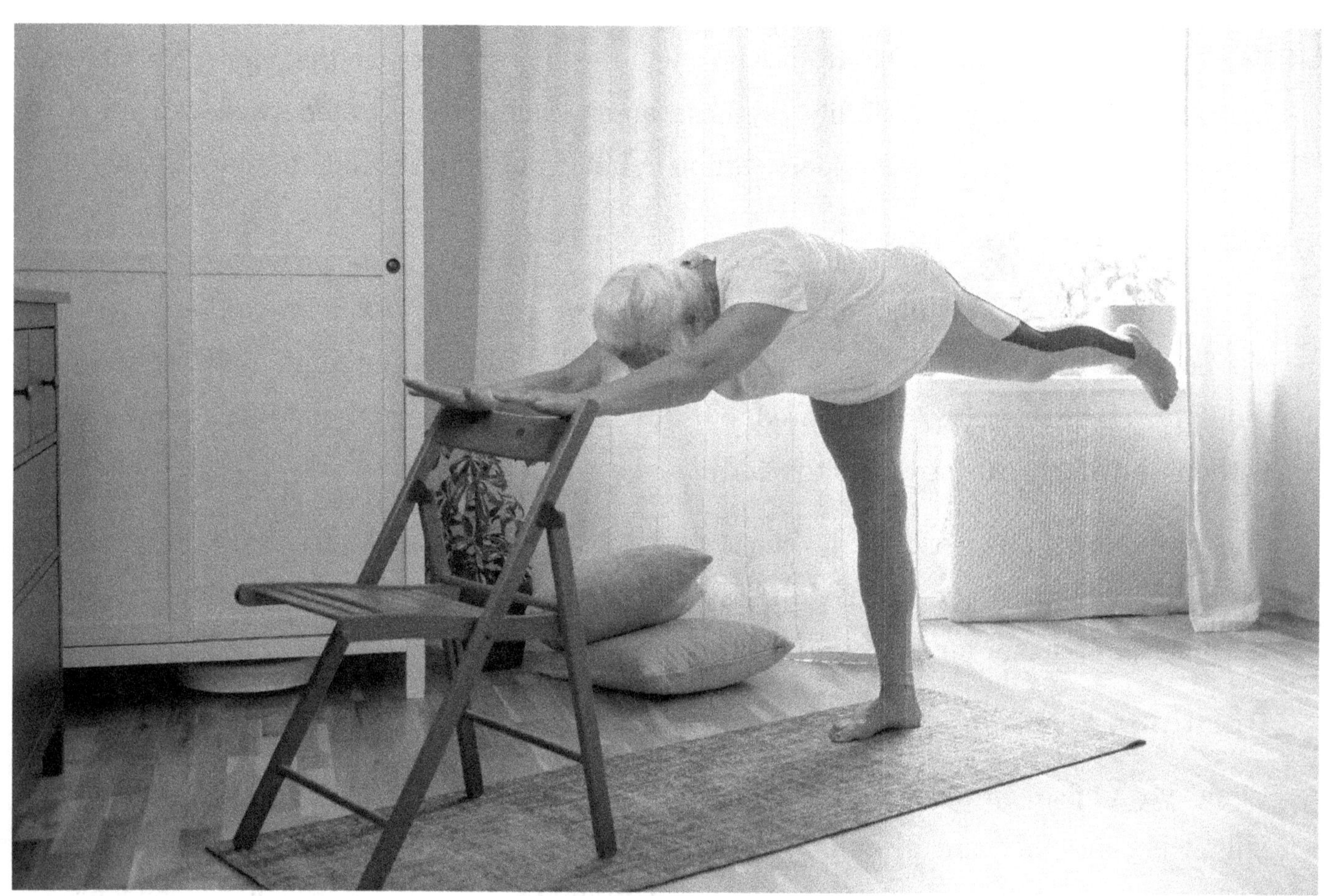

Building Strength and Balance

Building strength and balance is paramount for seniors, as these physical attributes are crucial for maintaining independence, preventing falls, and ensuring a high quality of life. Chair yoga, with its adaptability and accessibility, serves as a powerful tool in this regard, offering exercises that specifically target muscle strengthening and balance enhancement.

The Importance of Strength and Balance in Aging

As we age, our muscular strength and balance can naturally decline, making daily activities more challenging and increasing the risk of falls, which are a leading cause of injury among seniors. Building strength is not only about improving muscle mass but also about enhancing the functionality of the muscles, enabling better support for the joints and spine. Balance, on the other hand, is essential for performing everyday tasks safely, from walking to climbing stairs and even standing up from a seated position.

Chair Yoga's Approach to Strengthening and Balancing

Chair yoga addresses the need for strength and balance through a series of seated and standing poses that utilize the chair for support. This approach ensures safety while effectively challenging the body's muscles and balance systems.

Strengthening Through Resistance

One of the ways chair yoga builds strength is through the use of the body's own weight as resistance. For example, seated leg lifts not only improve the strength of the quadriceps but also engage the core muscles, vital for spine support and balance. Similarly, arm raises with or without the addition of light hand weights can strengthen the shoulders and upper back, areas crucial for daily activities that involve lifting or reaching.

Chair yoga also encourages the engagement of multiple muscle groups simultaneously, which not only builds strength but also simulates real-life movements where such coordination is essential. For instance, a chair-supported warrior pose strengthens the legs, opens the hips, and stretches the chest and shoulders, all while challenging balance and promoting functional muscle use.

Enhancing Balance with Focused Poses

Balance is enhanced in chair yoga through poses that require maintaining stability while changing the base of support or shifting the body's weight. For example, a seated or standing tree pose, where one foot is placed on the opposite leg while the arms reach upwards, challenges the body to maintain equilibrium, thereby improving balance.

Furthermore, chair yoga incorporates dynamic movements that mimic everyday activities, such as transitioning from sitting to standing. These movements not only build muscle strength but also train the body to maintain balance during motion, reducing the risk of falls.

The Role of Focus and Concentration

Chair yoga exercises for balance often require focus and concentration, which can further enhance the body's stability mechanisms. By concentrating on maintaining a specific pose or following a sequence of movements, seniors can improve their proprioception — the body's ability to sense its position in space. This heightened awareness is key to maintaining balance both during static poses and in motion.

The Synergistic Benefits of Strength and Balance Training

The combined focus on building strength and enhancing balance in chair yoga offers synergistic benefits. Improved muscle strength supports the body's joints and aids in maintaining proper posture, which is foundational for good balance. At the same time, practicing balance exercises enhances proprioception and coordination, reducing the risk of falls and injuries, and contributing to a sense of confidence and independence among seniors.

Incorporating chair yoga into a regular fitness routine can lead to significant improvements in both strength and balance. Seniors can expect not only to perform daily tasks more easily and safely but also to enjoy an overall enhancement in their quality of life. With each session of chair yoga, the journey towards greater mobility, stability, and independence continues, demonstrating that age is but a number when it comes to maintaining physical health and well-being.

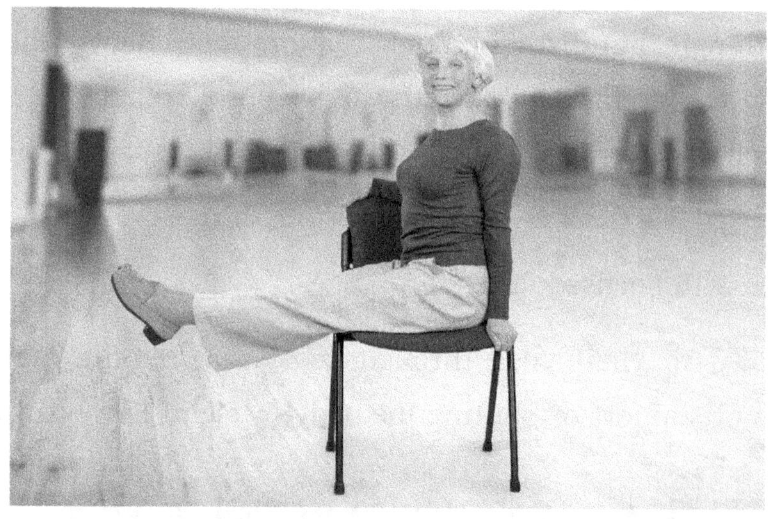

Reducing Stress and Improving Mental Health

Reducing stress and improving mental health are critical components of overall well-being, particularly for seniors who may face various life transitions and health challenges. Chair yoga offers a gentle yet effective way to address these aspects, emphasizing the mind-body connection and fostering a state of relaxation and mental clarity.

Understanding Stress and Mental Health in Seniors

For many seniors, the golden years bring not only wisdom but also an array of stressors such as health issues, loss of loved ones, changes in living situations, and concerns about independence and mobility. These stressors can have a significant impact on mental health, potentially leading to feelings of anxiety, depression, and isolation. Moreover, chronic stress can exacerbate physical health problems, creating a cycle that affects overall quality of life.

How Chair Yoga Addresses Stress and Mental Health

Chair yoga, with its focus on gentle movements, breathing techniques, and mindfulness, serves as a holistic approach to reducing stress and enhancing mental well-being. By engaging in chair yoga, seniors can tap into several mechanisms that help mitigate stress and improve mood.

Breathing Techniques for Relaxation

One of the foundational elements of chair yoga is the practice of controlled breathing, or pranayama. These breathing techniques can directly influence the body's stress response, shifting from the sympathetic nervous system's "fight or flight" mode to the parasympathetic nervous system's "rest and digest" state. Techniques such as deep diaphragmatic breathing, alternate nostril breathing, or simply focusing on slow, rhythmic breaths can help calm the mind, reduce anxiety, and foster a sense of inner peace.

Gentle Movements to Release Tension

Chair yoga incorporates a variety of seated and standing poses that are designed to gently stretch and mobilize the body. These movements can help release physical tension that is often held in key areas like the neck, shoulders, and back as a result of stress. By focusing on gentle stretching and mindful movement, participants can experience immediate relief from discomfort, leading to a more relaxed and comfortable state of being.

Mindfulness and Meditation for Mental Clarity

Mindfulness and meditation are integral parts of chair yoga, encouraging participants to bring their attention to the present moment. This practice can help break the cycle of stress-inducing thoughts and worries about the past or future. Through guided meditation, visualization, or simply maintaining a mindful awareness during yoga poses, seniors can cultivate a state of mental clarity, reduce rumination, and improve their ability to cope with stress.

The Role of Community and Connection

Participating in chair yoga, whether in a group setting or through virtual classes, can also provide a sense of community and connection. For seniors, especially those who may feel isolated, this social aspect of chair yoga can be incredibly beneficial. Sharing experiences, encouragement, and support with others can bolster feelings of belonging and improve overall mental health.

The Comprehensive Benefits of Chair Yoga for Mental Well-Being

By addressing stress reduction, relaxation, and mental clarity in an accessible and gentle manner, chair yoga offers seniors a powerful tool for improving mental health. The cumulative effect of regular practice can lead to significant improvements in mood, a reduction in symptoms of anxiety and depression, and an enhanced sense of well-being. As seniors incorporate chair yoga into their lives, they not only reclaim their physical independence but also embrace a more empowered and joyful state of mind.

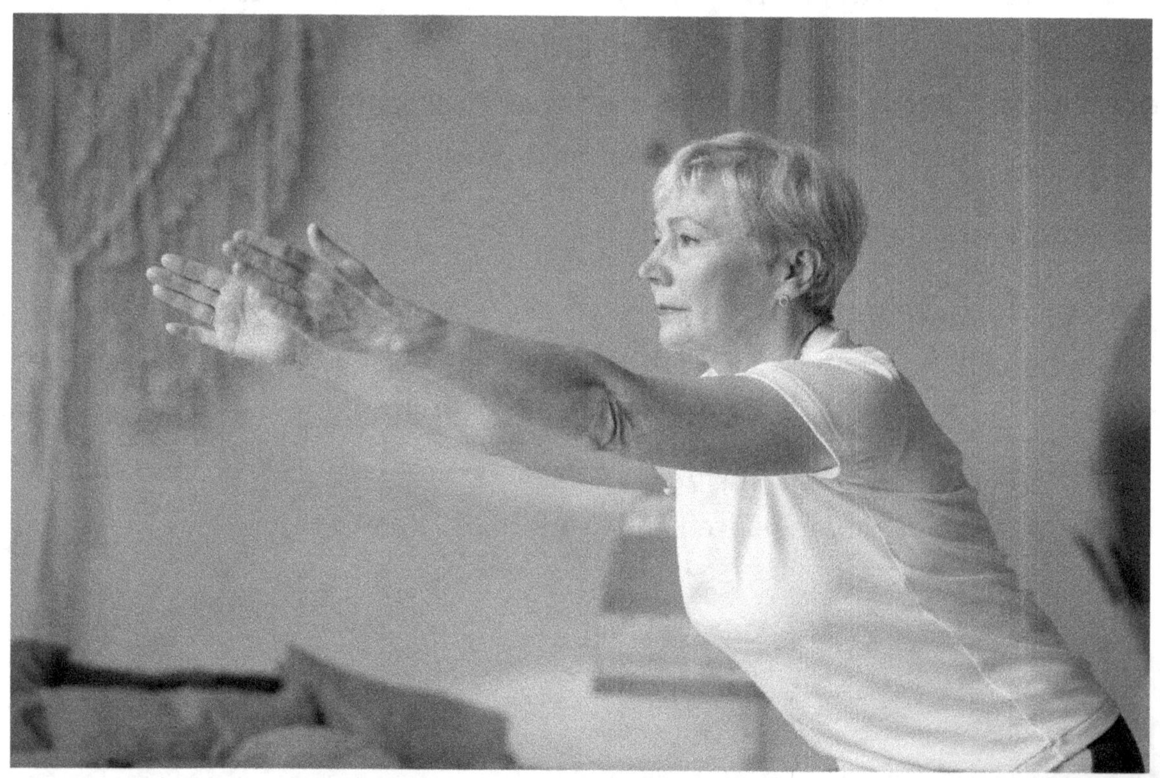

Promoting Independence and Quality of Life

Promoting independence and enhancing the quality of life are fundamental goals for seniors seeking to maintain a vibrant, fulfilling lifestyle as they age. Chair yoga emerges as a key ally in this quest, offering a multifaceted approach to preserving autonomy and enriching daily living. This gentle form of exercise not only caters to physical well-being but also fortifies the emotional and mental resilience necessary for seniors to navigate the complexities of aging with grace and dignity.

Fostering Physical Autonomy

The capacity for independent movement is at the heart of personal freedom for seniors. The loss of this capability can significantly impact one's quality of life, leading to reliance on caregivers for basic activities such as walking, bending, or even sitting and standing. Chair yoga addresses these concerns head-on by focusing on strengthening muscles, enhancing flexibility, and improving balance. Through targeted exercises, seniors can regain and maintain the muscle strength and joint mobility essential for everyday tasks, thus preserving their independence.

Specific poses in chair yoga are designed to mimic daily movements, such as reaching for objects on a high shelf or bending down to tie a shoe, ensuring that practice translates directly into real-world benefits. Improved balance, a direct outcome of regular chair yoga practice, significantly reduces the risk of falls—a major concern for the elderly—further supporting an autonomous lifestyle.

Enhancing Emotional Well-Being

Independence is not solely a physical matter; it encompasses the ability to manage one's emotional well-being. Chair yoga offers a holistic approach to health that includes stress reduction, mindfulness, and the cultivation of a positive outlook. The meditative aspects of yoga encourage practitioners to find peace and contentment within themselves, fostering a sense of emotional autonomy. This inner resilience is crucial for facing age-related challenges with confidence and grace, rather than fear and dependency.

Social Engagement and Community

Quality of life is profoundly influenced by social connections and a sense of belonging. Chair yoga classes, whether held in community centers, online, or in senior living facilities, provide valuable opportunities for social interaction. These communal settings not only enhance the physical benefits of yoga practice but also fulfill the human need for companionship and mutual support. Engaging with peers in a positive, health-oriented activity fosters a sense of community that can combat feelings of isolation and loneliness among seniors.

Intellectual Stimulation and Lifelong Learning

Engaging in chair yoga also offers cognitive benefits, contributing to a senior's quality of life by providing opportunities for learning and mental engagement. Mastering new poses, understanding the principles of yoga, and exploring the mind-body connection stimulate the brain and encourage a mindset of lifelong learning and curiosity. This intellectual engagement is essential for maintaining cognitive health and fostering a sense of personal growth and fulfillment at any age.

A Path to Empowered Aging

Ultimately, chair yoga empowers seniors to take control of their health and well-being. By providing tools for physical maintenance, emotional resilience, social connection, and intellectual engagement, chair yoga lays the foundation for a high quality of life and independence. Seniors who embrace chair yoga find themselves not merely aging but aging gracefully, with an enhanced capacity to enjoy each day to its fullest, engage with their communities, and celebrate the autonomy that defines a life well-lived.

Conclusion

In conclusion, through chair yoga, seniors are equipped with the tools necessary to combat the physical and mental challenges that come with aging, transforming these years into a period of growth, joy, and independence.

The journey through chair yoga is one of rediscovery — rediscovering the strength within one's body, the peace within one's mind, and the joy within one's spirit. It's about breaking the chains of physical limitations and societal expectations to carve out a path of wellness that is both fulfilling and sustainable. Chair yoga provides the means to enhance mobility, flexibility, and balance, reducing the risk of falls and improving overall physical health. But its benefits extend far beyond the physical realm, offering a sanctuary for the mind and a balm for the soul.

By reducing stress and improving mental health, chair yoga opens the door to a life less burdened by anxiety and more enriched by moments of peace and mindfulness. It fosters a sense of community and belonging, reminding seniors that they are not alone in their journey. Every pose, every breath, and every moment of mindfulness is a step toward reclaiming not just physical independence, but the joy of movement and the freedom to live life on one's own terms.

As we look toward the future, Chair Yoga Revolution stands as a testament to the timeless nature of yoga and its adaptability to meet the needs of seniors today. It challenges the narrative of aging as a decline, offering instead a vision of aging as an opportunity for continued growth, learning, and happiness. This guide is a call to action for seniors to embrace chair yoga as a way to enhance their quality of life, promote independence, and age with dignity and strength.

In embracing chair yoga, seniors are not just practicing a form of exercise; they are joining a revolution — a movement toward a society where aging is celebrated, where seniors are empowered to lead active and engaged lives, and where the golden years are truly golden. Let Chair Yoga Revolution be your companion on this journey, guiding you through each pose, each breath, and each step toward a healthier, happier, and more independent you.

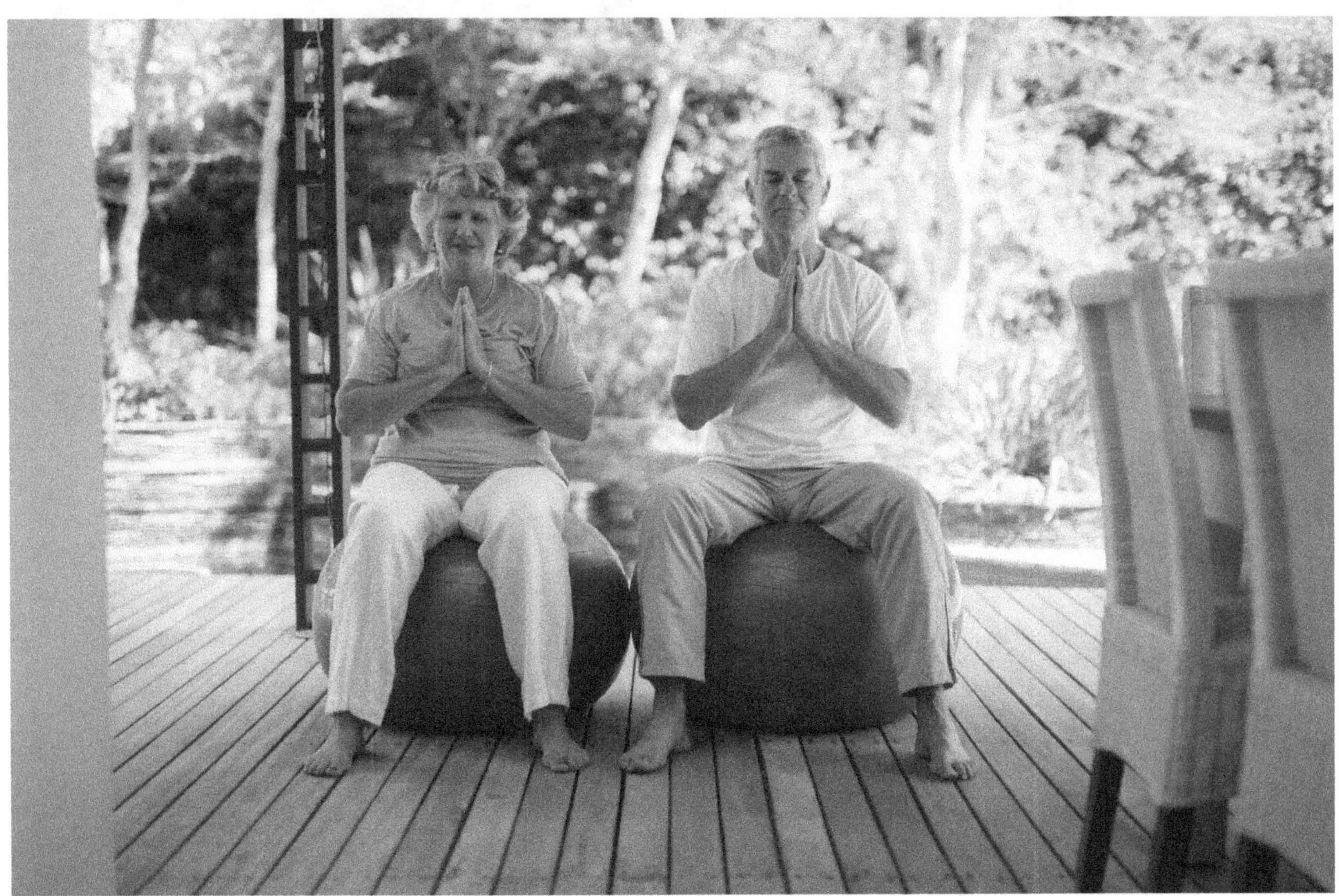

Chapter 3:

Getting Started with Chair Yoga

Chair yoga offers a gentle form of yoga that is performed sitting on a chair or standing using a chair for support. This makes it perfect for seniors or anyone with mobility issues, chronic pain, or the desire to maintain independence. The key to beginning your chair yoga journey is understanding its benefits and knowing how to start safely.

Identifying Personal Goals (with Examples)

When embarking on a chair yoga journey, setting personal goals is a crucial step. These goals give you direction, motivate you to stay on track, and provide a sense of accomplishment as you progress. Here's how to identify your personal goals for chair yoga, along with examples to inspire you:

Step 1: Reflect on Your Needs and Desires

Begin by considering what you wish to achieve through chair yoga. Is it physical wellness, mental clarity, or perhaps a combination of both? Reflecting on your current health status, daily challenges, and long-term aspirations can help clarify your objectives.

Example Goals:

1. Improving Flexibility: You might find certain daily tasks, like bending to tie your shoes or reaching for items on a high shelf, have become challenging. A goal could be to enhance your flexibility, making these tasks easier and reducing discomfort.

2. Enhancing Balance: Perhaps you've noticed a slight unsteadiness while walking or standing. Setting a goal to improve your balance can help reduce the risk of falls, a common concern for seniors, thereby increasing your confidence in moving freely.

3. Building Strength: Losing muscle mass and strength can affect your ability to perform everyday activities. A goal could involve strengthening key muscle groups to support your mobility and independence.

4. Reducing Stress: If you're experiencing stress or anxiety, a goal might be to utilize chair yoga as a tool for relaxation, harnessing breathing exercises and meditation to foster a sense of calm.

5. Alleviating Chronic Pain: For those dealing with chronic pain, such as arthritis or back pain, a goal could be to mitigate discomfort through gentle movements and stretches tailored to your condition.

Step 2: Make Your Goals Specific and Achievable

Once you've identified your broad objectives, refine them into specific, achievable goals. This approach ensures your goals are clear and measurable, providing a tangible path to follow.

Refining Your Goals:

Instead of simply aiming to "improve flexibility," set a goal to "perform a seated forward bend without discomfort within three months."

Rather than a general desire to "reduce stress," aim to "practice chair yoga breathing exercises for 10 minutes daily, feeling more relaxed and focused afterward."

Step 3: Break Down Your Goals into Actionable Steps

With your specific goals in mind, outline the steps needed to achieve them. This might involve scheduling regular chair yoga sessions, focusing on particular poses or exercises, and tracking your progress over time.

Actionable Steps Examples:

For improving flexibility, dedicate the first 5 minutes of each session to stretches that target your hamstrings and back.

To enhance balance, incorporate standing poses using the chair for support twice a week, gradually increasing the duration as your stability improves.

For strength building, include chair yoga exercises that engage your arms, legs, and core, gradually incorporating light weights or resistance bands.

Step 4: Regularly Review and Adjust Your Goals

As you progress in your chair yoga practice, take time to review your goals. Celebrate the milestones you've achieved, and if necessary, adjust your goals to reflect your current abilities and aspirations. This ongoing process ensures your chair yoga practice continues to meet your evolving needs.

Identifying personal goals for chair yoga is a deeply personal process that requires introspection and honesty. By setting specific, achievable objectives, you create a roadmap for your journey towards improved well-being. Remember, the beauty of chair yoga lies in its adaptability; it can be tailored to meet your unique needs and aspirations, making it a powerful ally in your pursuit of a healthier, more fulfilling life.

Step-by-Step Actions

1. Choose the Right Chair:

The journey into Chair Yoga begins with the selection of a suitable chair. Opt for a sturdy chair that doesn't have wheels, ensuring it won't slip or move during your practice. The chair should allow your feet to rest comfortably on the ground, with knees at a 90-degree angle. This position facilitates proper posture and stability during exercises.

2. Create a Safe Space:

Your practice area should be your sanctuary. Clear the space around your chair of any potential hazards that could cause tripping or distraction. If you're on a smooth surface, placing a non-slip yoga mat under your chair can add an extra layer of security. Adequate lighting and a peaceful atmosphere will also enhance your focus and overall experience.

3. Gather Equipment:

While the essence of Chair Yoga lies in its simplicity, a few items can augment your practice. A yoga mat provides a stable surface for your chair, a water bottle keeps you hydrated, and comfortable clothing allows unrestricted movement. Additionally, consider having a cushion for extra support and a blanket for warmth during relaxation phases.

4. Start with Breathing:

Breathing is the cornerstone of yoga. Initiate each session with a few minutes dedicated to deep, mindful breathing. This practice helps center your thoughts, oxygenates your body, and prepares you for physical activity. It sets the tone for a session that is as much about mental well-being as it is about physical health.

5. Follow a Structured Routine:

A balanced session includes a warm-up, the main sequence, and a cool-down. Begin with gentle stretches to awaken the body. Gradually move into a series of poses designed to strengthen muscles and improve balance. Conclude with a period of relaxation and deep breathing, allowing your body to assimilate the benefits of your practice.

For Women:

Women can greatly benefit from Chair Yoga, especially with poses that target the pelvic floor, enhancing both strength and flexibility. This focus can aid in managing symptoms of menopause and strengthening the core, vital for women's health as they age.

For Those New to Exercise:

If exercise hasn't been a part of your routine, Chair Yoga is a welcoming gateway. Start with foundational poses, appreciating the form and feeling each movement brings. It's not about perfection but progression. Celebrate each small achievement, building confidence and capability at your own pace.

For People with Specific Health Concerns:

Chair Yoga is inclusive, offering modifications to accommodate various health conditions. If arthritis is a concern, focus on gentle joint movements. For back pain, emphasize core strengthening and spine-supporting poses. The key is to listen to your body, never pushing into pain, and using props like cushions for added support and comfort.

This approach ensures Chair Yoga is accessible and rewarding for everyone, regardless of age, health status, or fitness level. By tailoring the practice to individual needs and goals, it becomes a powerful tool for enhancing quality of life.

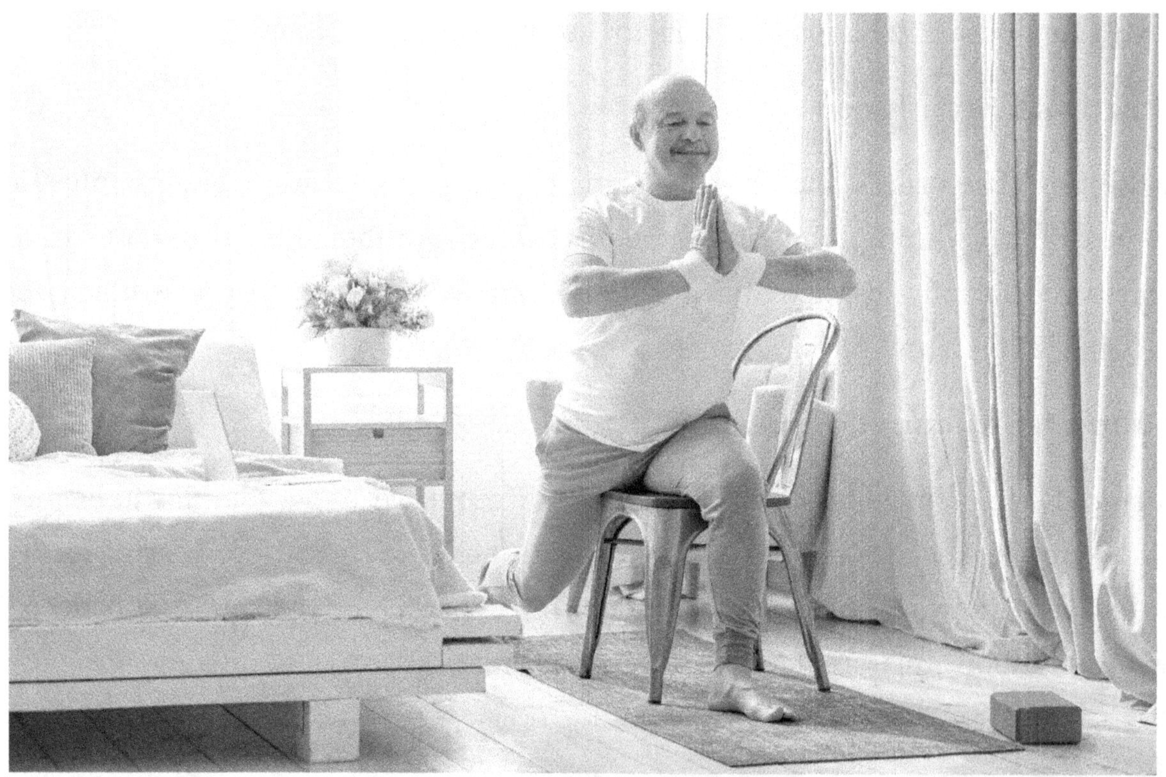

Chapter 4:

Chair Yoga Poses and Exercises

Welcome to a journey of rejuvenation, empowerment, and self-discovery through Chair Yoga, a practice that has revolutionized the way we approach wellness in our senior years. This chapter serves as your gateway to a world where mobility limitations and chronic pain are not barriers to experiencing the profound benefits of yoga. Instead, they are touchstones for adapting and embracing a practice that meets you exactly where you are.

Chair Yoga is not merely a subset of yoga; it is a comprehensive approach tailored specifically for seniors seeking to enhance their quality of life. It acknowledges the unique challenges faced by older adults, offering a gentle yet effective path to maintaining and improving physical health, mental clarity, and emotional well-being. Through the step-by-step guide outlined in this chapter, you will discover how to embark on this practice safely, confidently, and with joy.

The essence of Chair Yoga lies in its accessibility. Whether you are contending with reduced mobility, managing chronic pain, or simply looking for a safe way to stay active, chair yoga opens the door to numerous possibilities for health and wellness. It allows you to engage in a variety of yoga poses and exercises specifically adapted to be performed with the aid of a chair, ensuring stability and support as you stretch, strengthen, and soothe your body and mind.

This chapter aims to demystify the practice of chair yoga, making it approachable for all seniors, regardless of their fitness level, experience with yoga, or health conditions. Here, you will find detailed instructions on a range of poses and exercises—from gentle stretches that enhance flexibility and mobility to strength-building movements that foster balance and endurance. Each exercise is presented with clear, step-by-step actions, accompanied by examples and variations to cater to different needs and preferences.

Moreover, this guide recognizes the diverse audience it serves, including women seeking pelvic floor strengthening, individuals new to exercise, and those with specific health concerns such as arthritis or back pain. By providing different angles and variations, this chapter ensures that everyone can find a way to engage with chair yoga in a manner that respects their body's unique needs and enhances their overall well-being.

Beyond the physical benefits, chair yoga offers profound mental and emotional advantages. Through breathing exercises, mindfulness practices, and the nurturing of a supportive community, chair yoga promotes stress reduction, mental clarity, and a sense of peace and contentment. It champions the idea that aging can be an empowering journey of maintaining independence, embracing joy, and discovering new strengths.

As you turn the pages of this chapter, allow yourself to be open to the transformative potential of chair yoga. Herein lies an opportunity to not only revitalize your body but to also nourish your mind and spirit. Embrace this chance to revolutionize your approach to aging, enhancing your mobility, strength, and independence, one pose at a time.

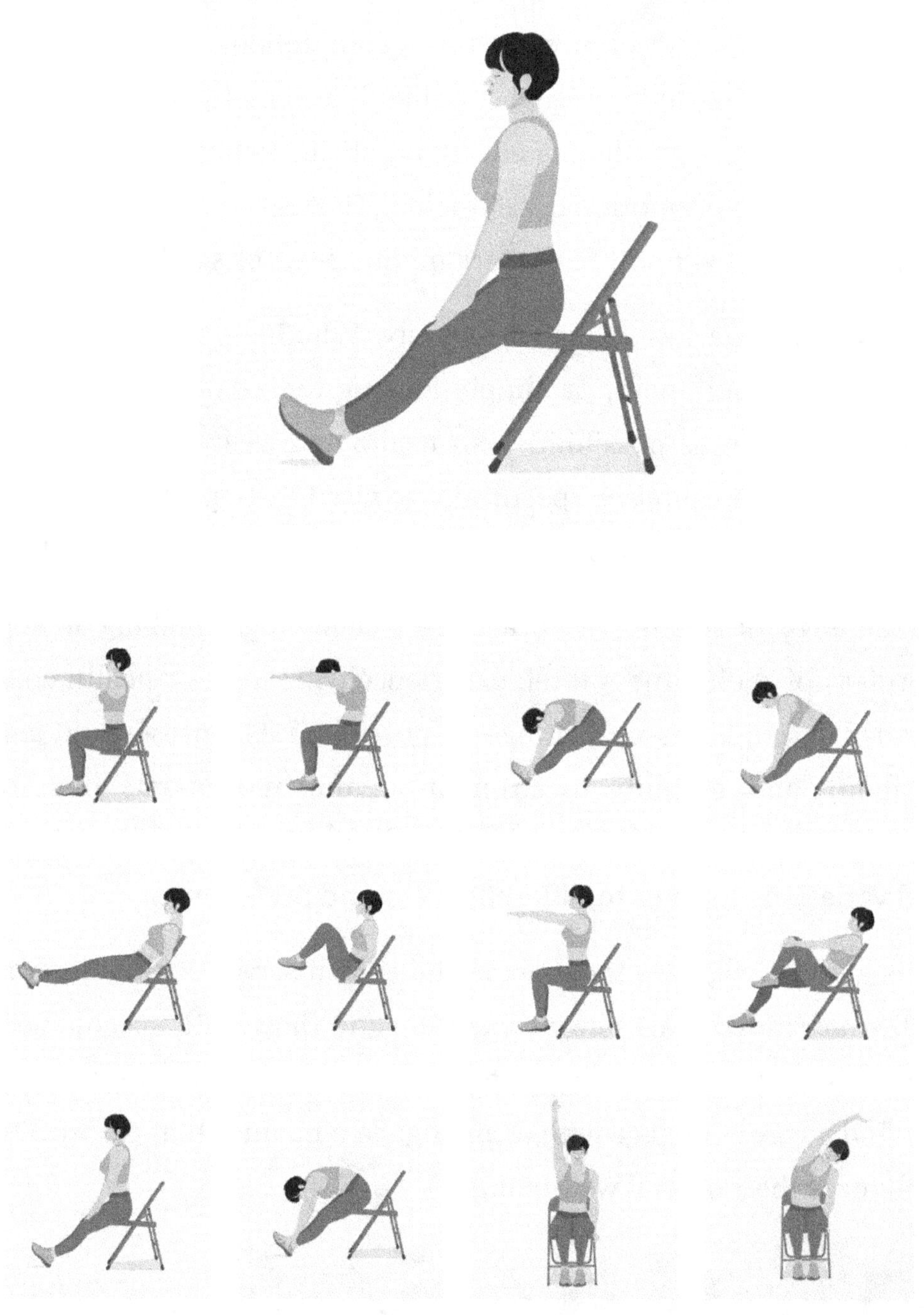

Warm-Up Exercises for Chair Yoga

Before diving into the core chair yoga poses that build strength, enhance flexibility, and promote balance, it's crucial to begin with a proper warm-up. Warm-up exercises gently prepare the body for physical activity, reducing the risk of injury and making your yoga practice more effective. For seniors, individuals with osteoarthritis, chronic pain, balance issues, cardiovascular health concerns, flexibility and range of motion challenges, or those seeking mental wellbeing, these exercises are designed to address your specific needs, ensuring a safe and enjoyable yoga experience.

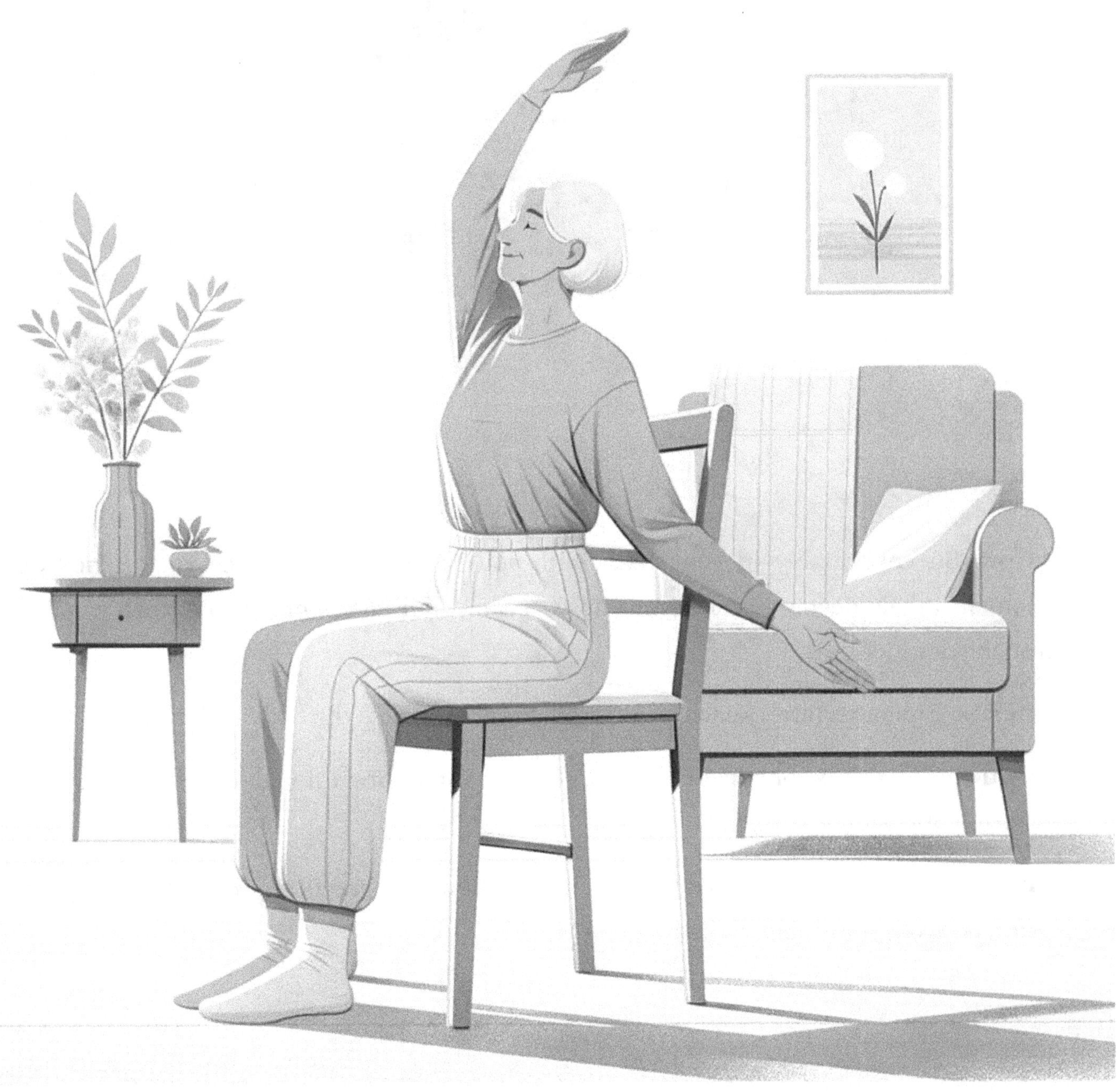

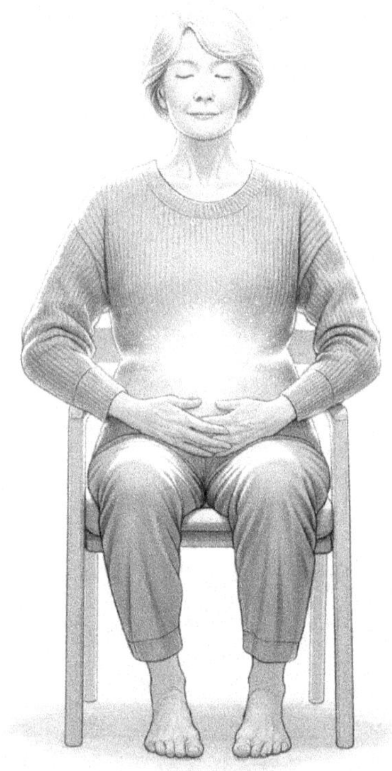

Action: Sit comfortably in your chair with your back straight. Place your hands on your abdomen. Inhale deeply through your nose, feeling your abdomen expand, then exhale slowly through your mouth.

Benefits: Enhances lung capacity, calms the mind, prepares the body for exercise.

Common Mistakes: Shallow breathing. Ensure you're breathing deeply into your abdomen, not just your chest.

Supplementary Content: Pair this with mindfulness practice by focusing fully on your breath, clearing your mind of distractions.

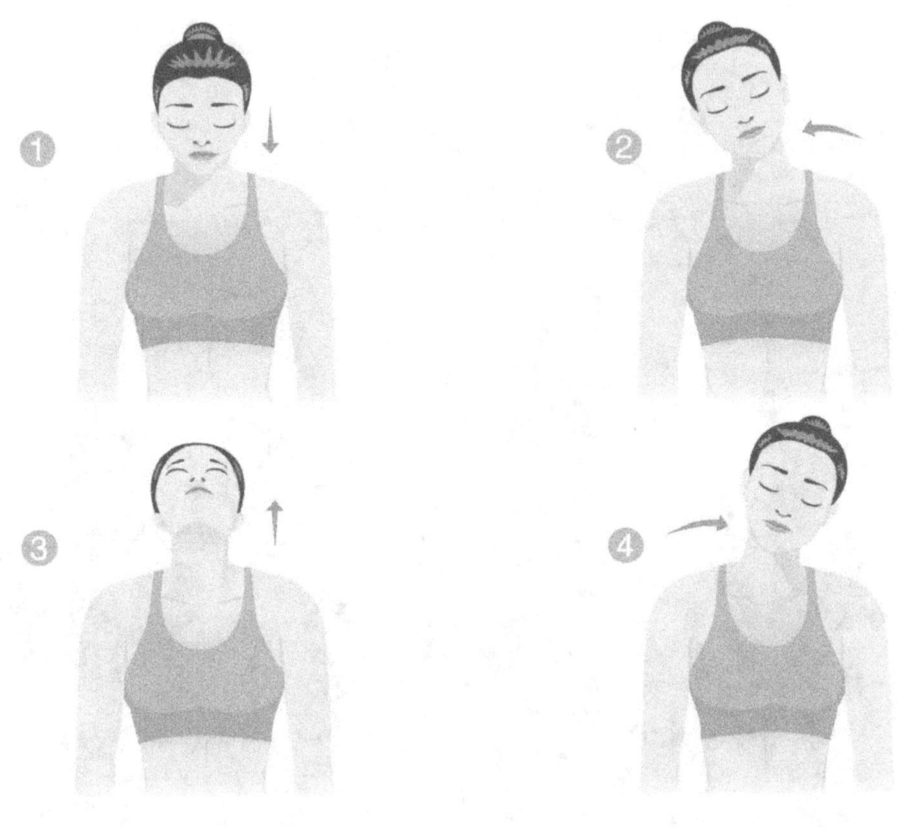

Action: Gently lower your chin to your chest, then slowly roll your head to one side, back, to the other side, and down, creating a smooth circular motion. Repeat for the shoulders by rolling them forwards and backwards.

Benefits: Releases tension in the neck and shoulders, improves flexibility.

Common Mistakes: Rushing the movements. Move slowly to avoid dizziness and maximize the release of tension.

Supplementary Content: Combine with a breathing technique, inhaling as you move up and exhaling as you move down.

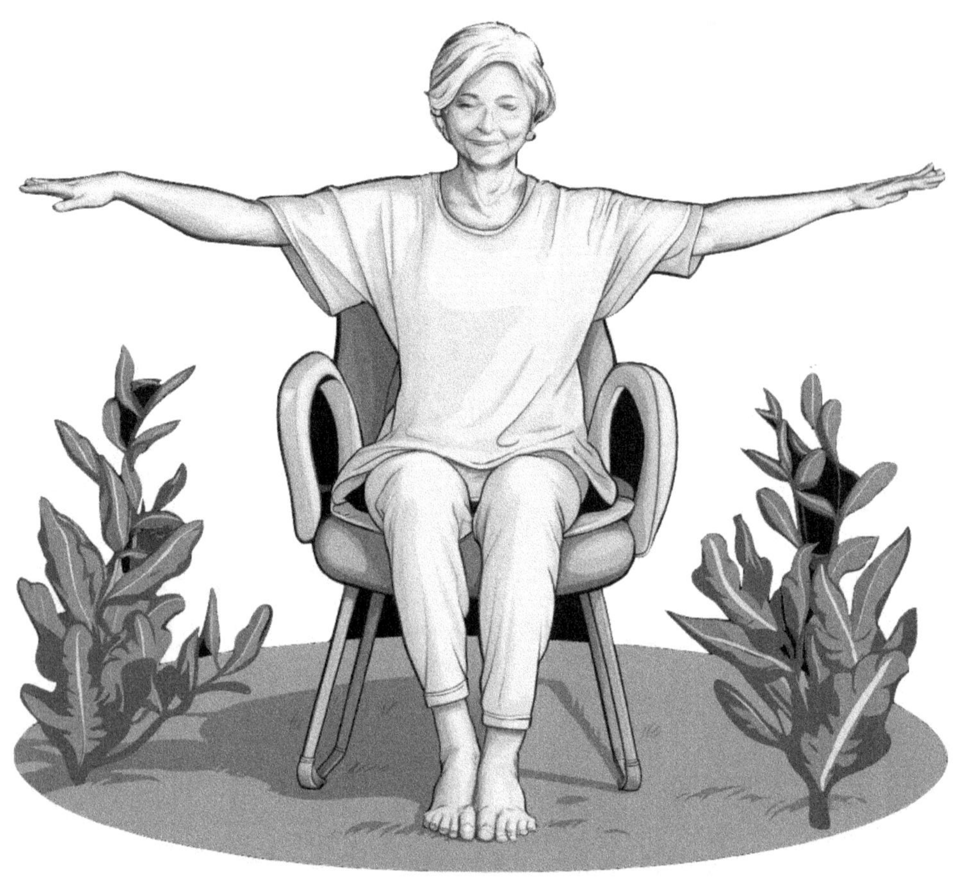

Action: With palms facing forward, breathe in and lift your arms to the side until they are at shoulder height, then gently lower them while exhaling.

Benefits: Improves circulation, builds shoulder flexibility.

Common Mistakes: Lifting shoulders towards the ears. Keep your shoulders relaxed.

Supplementary Content: Visualize drawing energy up as you lift your arms and releasing it as you lower them, fostering a sense of energy flow.

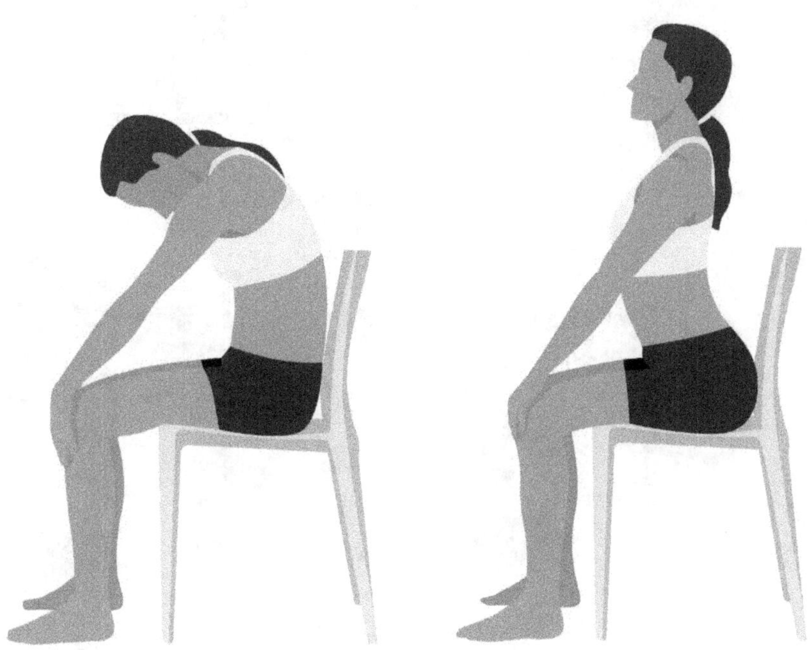

Action: Place your hands on your knees. Inhale, arch your back and look up towards the ceiling (Cow). Exhale, round your spine, tucking your chin to your chest (Cat).

Benefits: Increases spine flexibility, stimulates the digestive tract.

Common Mistakes: Forgetting to sync breath with movement. Remember, the movement extends from your tailbone to your neck.

Supplementary Content: Think about releasing any negative emotions on the exhale and inviting positivity on the inhale.

Seated Marching

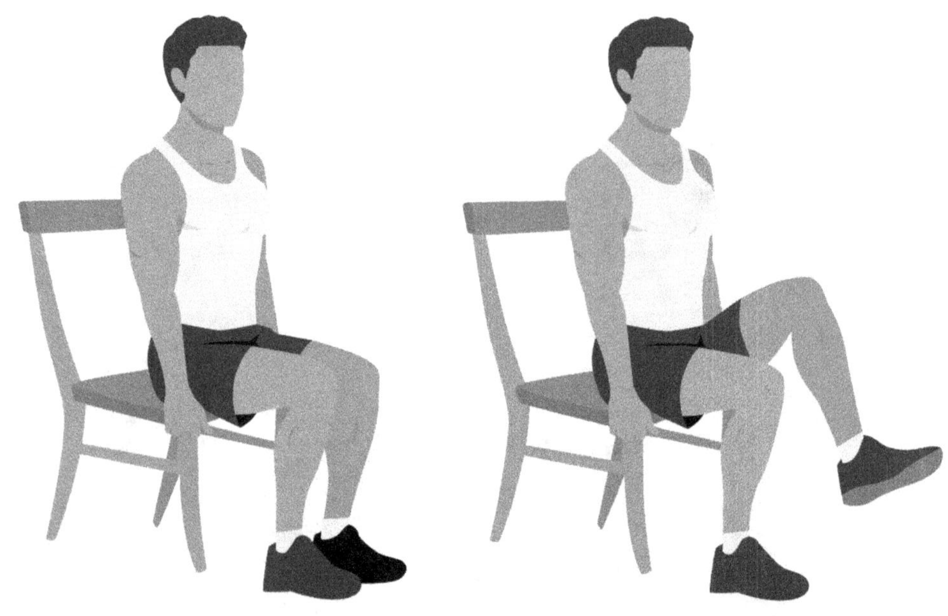

Action: Hold onto the sides of the chair. Lift your right knee as high as comfortable, then lower it and repeat with the left knee, as if marching in place.

Benefits: Warms up the lower body, enhances hip mobility.

Common Mistakes: Leaning back as you lift your legs. Maintain an upright posture.

Supplementary Content: Focus on engaging your core as you lift each knee to build stability.

Warm-up exercises are an essential foundation of your chair yoga practice, preparing your body and mind for the session ahead. By incorporating these exercises into your routine, you address specific health concerns while setting the stage for a fulfilling and beneficial yoga experience. Remember, the key to a successful practice lies in listening to your body and moving at a pace that feels right for you.

Developing a Progress Log or Journal

To engage deeply with the practice of chair yoga and to maximize its benefits, keeping a progress log or journal is a highly effective strategy. This simple yet profound habit can transform your yoga journey, offering insights into your physical and emotional evolution. Below, we expand on how to incorporate this practice into your daily routine, making each session of chair yoga more meaningful and personalized.

1. **Choosing Your Medium:**

   Decide whether you prefer a traditional notebook, a digital app, or a simple document on your computer. The key is convenience and regular access.

2. **Structuring Your Entries**:

   Date each session for reference

   Before the Session: Note any physical sensations, emotional states, or specific areas of tightness or discomfort in your body. This initial observation sets a baseline for your practice.

   After the Session: Reflect on changes in your physical sensations, emotional state, and areas of improvement in flexibility or mobility. Note any poses that were challenging or particularly beneficial.

3. **Tracking Physical Improvements**:

   Record any increases in flexibility, such as being able to reach further in a forward bend or experiencing less discomfort in a particular pose.

   Note improvements in balance and strength, like holding a pose longer without support or feeling more stable in standing exercises.

4. **Observing Emotional and Mental Changes**:

   Reflect on changes in your stress levels, mood, and overall mental clarity. Chair yoga not only benefits the body but also significantly impacts mental health.

   Document moments of mindfulness or increased body awareness experienced during your practice.

5. **Setting Goals and Celebrating Achievements**:

   Use your journal to set short-term and long-term goals for your chair yoga practice. Goals can range from improving flexibility in a specific area to integrating more mindfulness into each session.

   Celebrate milestones, no matter how small, to stay motivated. Recognizing your progress is crucial for maintaining enthusiasm and dedication to your practice.

6. **Enhancing Mindfulness and Connection**:

   Before closing your journal, take a moment to express gratitude for your body's capabilities and for the opportunity to engage in your practice. This fosters a deeper connection to your yoga journey and encourages a positive mindset.

7. **Review and Reflect**:

   Periodically review your journal entries to observe your journey over time. This can provide valuable insights into patterns in your physical or emotional wellbeing and guide future practice.

The Benefits of Keeping a Progress Log

Personalized Feedback: Your journal becomes a personalized feedback loop, helping you tailor your chair yoga practice to your evolving needs.

Enhanced Awareness: Regularly documenting your experiences enhances mindfulness, making you more attuned to the subtle changes in your body and mind.

Motivation: Seeing your progress in black and white can be incredibly motivating, encouraging you to continue with your practice.

Holistic View: A journal offers a holistic view of your practice, reminding you that yoga benefits not just the body, but also the mind and spirit.

By integrating a progress log or journal into your chair yoga routine, you create a rich, personalized narrative of your journey towards enhanced mobility, strength, and independence. This practice not only tracks your physical improvements but also deepens your mindfulness and connection to your body, enriching your overall yoga experience.

CLAIM

YOUR BONUS

NOW

and stay tuned for news, advices and additional contents

Chapter 5:

Chair Yoga Poses for Strength

Upper Body Strengthening

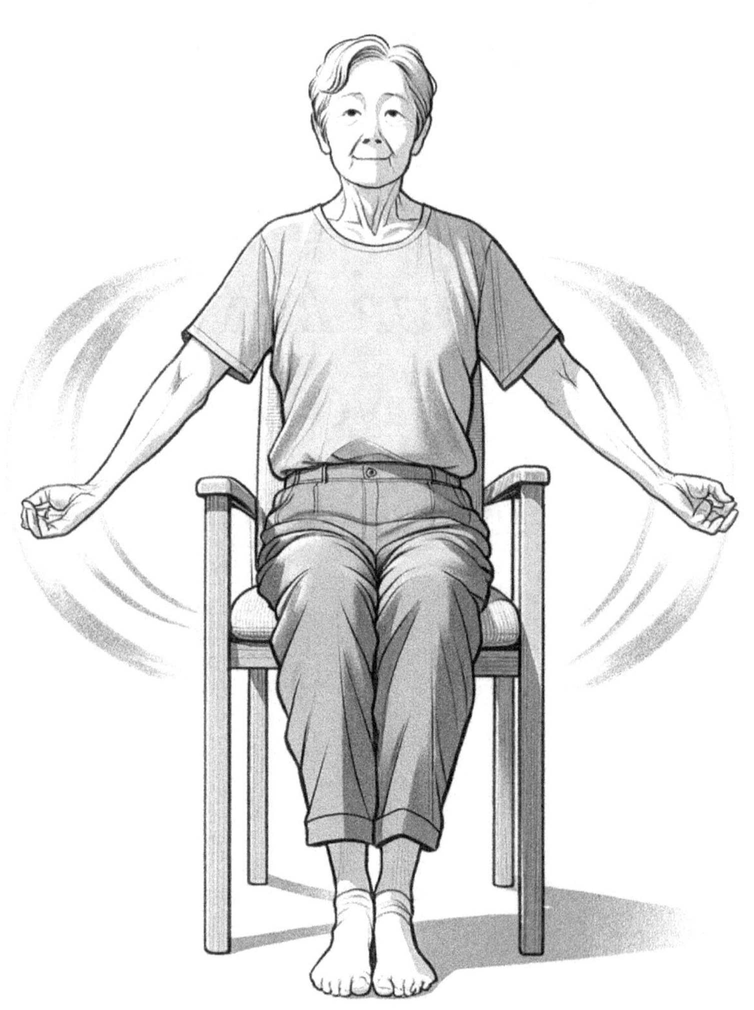

As we age, maintaining mobility and strength in our shoulders is crucial for performing daily activities with ease. Arm circles, a simple yet effective chair yoga exercise, offer a way to gently work the shoulder joints and muscles, enhancing flexibility and reducing stiffness. This chapter will guide you through the correct execution of arm circles, explore their benefits, highlight common mistakes, and suggest variations to accommodate different needs.

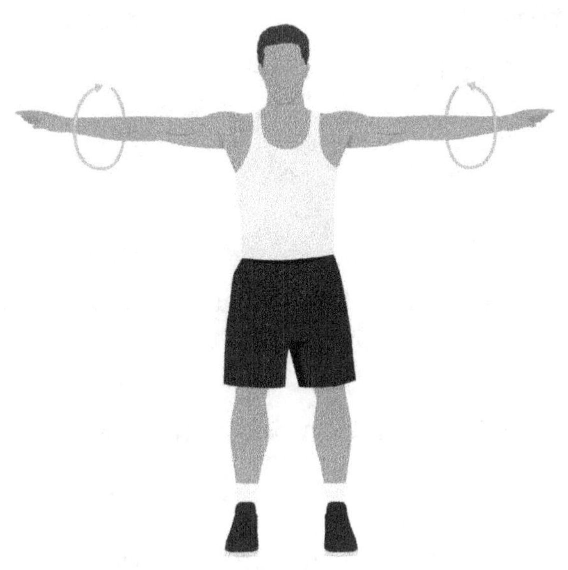

Actions

Sit Comfortably: Begin by sitting in a sturdy, armless chair with your feet flat on the ground, ensuring your back is straight but not stiff.

Position Your Arms: Extend your arms straight out to the sides at shoulder height, palms facing down.

Perform the Circles: Slowly start to make small circles with your arms, gradually increasing the size of the circles as you become more comfortable.

Reverse Direction: After completing 10-15 circles, reverse the direction for the same number of repetitions.

Cool Down: Lower your arms gently and shake them out to release any tension.

Benefits

Improved Shoulder Mobility: Regular practice helps to increase the range of motion in the shoulders.

Strengthens Shoulder Muscles: Arm circles engage the deltoids, rotator cuffs, and supporting shoulder girdle muscles, enhancing overall shoulder strength.

Reduces Stiffness: This exercise can alleviate stiffness and pain in the shoulder area, common in seniors.

Promotes Better Posture: Strengthening shoulder muscles contributes to better posture, reducing the risk of back and neck pain.

Common Mistakes

Overextending: Extending the arms too far or performing circles too quickly can strain the shoulder muscles.

Holding Breath: Forgetting to breathe smoothly throughout the exercise can increase tension in the shoulders.

Ignoring Pain: Continuing the exercise despite experiencing pain can lead to injuries. Always listen to your body and stop if discomfort occurs.

Variations

Seated with Support: For individuals with severe mobility issues or balance concerns, performing arm circles while seated against the back of the chair provides additional support.

Standing with Chair Assistance: Standing behind the chair and holding onto the backrest with one hand while performing arm circles with the other arm adds a balance challenge.

Adjusting Arm Height: For those with limited shoulder mobility, lowering the arms to a more comfortable height can make the exercise more accessible.

The Overhead Stretch is a fundamental chair yoga exercise that targets the upper body, promoting flexibility, releasing tension, and enhancing overall vitality. This chapter provides a step-by-step guide to performing the Overhead Stretch safely and effectively, highlighting its benefits for seniors with varying levels of mobility and offering variations to accommodate everyone.

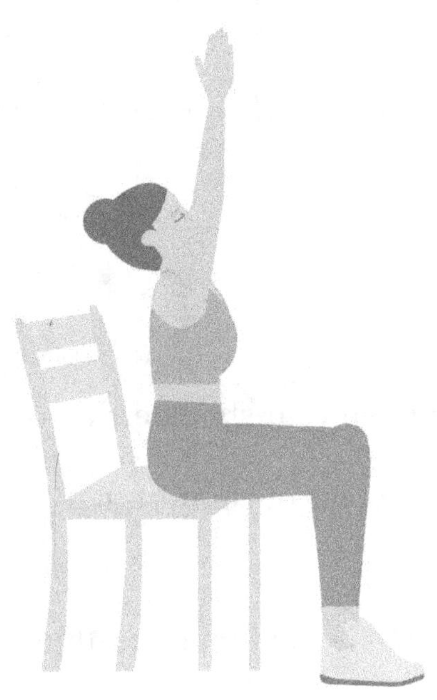

Actions

Start in a Seated Position: Sit in a sturdy, armless chair with your feet flat on the floor, spine straight, and shoulders relaxed.

Initiate the Stretch: Inhale deeply, and on the exhale, slowly raise your arms overhead, either keeping them parallel or clasping your hands together.

Deepen the Stretch: With your arms overhead, gently reach higher as if trying to touch the ceiling, keeping your shoulders down away from your ears. Hold for a few breaths.

Side Bends (Optional): For an added stretch, gently lean to one side, hold for a breath, come back to the center, and then lean to the other side.

Conclude the Exercise: Slowly lower your arms back down on an exhale, noticing the sensation of release in your shoulders and arms.

Benefits

Improves Upper Body Flexibility: Regular practice stretches the shoulders, arms, and torso, enhancing flexibility.

Reduces Tension and Stiffness: Helps alleviate tension in the upper back, neck, and shoulders.

Encourages Deep Breathing: The upward movement promotes fuller, deeper breaths, improving lung capacity.

Boosts Energy Levels: Invigorates the body and can increase alertness, making it an excellent morning exercise.

Common Mistakes

Raising Shoulders to Ears: Keep your shoulders relaxed to avoid tension in the neck.

Overstretching: Stretch to the point of comfort, not pain. Overstretching can lead to muscle strain.

Holding Breath: Maintain a steady, rhythmic breathing pattern throughout the stretch.

Variations

With a Towel: Holding a towel between your hands as you raise them overhead can help maintain arm alignment and provide a gentle, controlled stretch.

Seated or Standing: While traditionally performed seated, this stretch can also be done standing for those seeking a balance challenge.

Arm Width Adjustment: Altering the distance between your arms can change the stretch intensity. Closer arms intensify the stretch, while wider arms reduce intensity.

The Side Shoulder Stretch is a gentle yet effective chair yoga exercise tailored for seniors to relieve shoulder tension, enhance mobility, and contribute to overall upper body comfort. This chapter delivers a detailed guide for performing the Side Shoulder Stretch, underscoring its benefits, especially for seniors grappling with chronic pain, limited mobility, and the quest for independence.

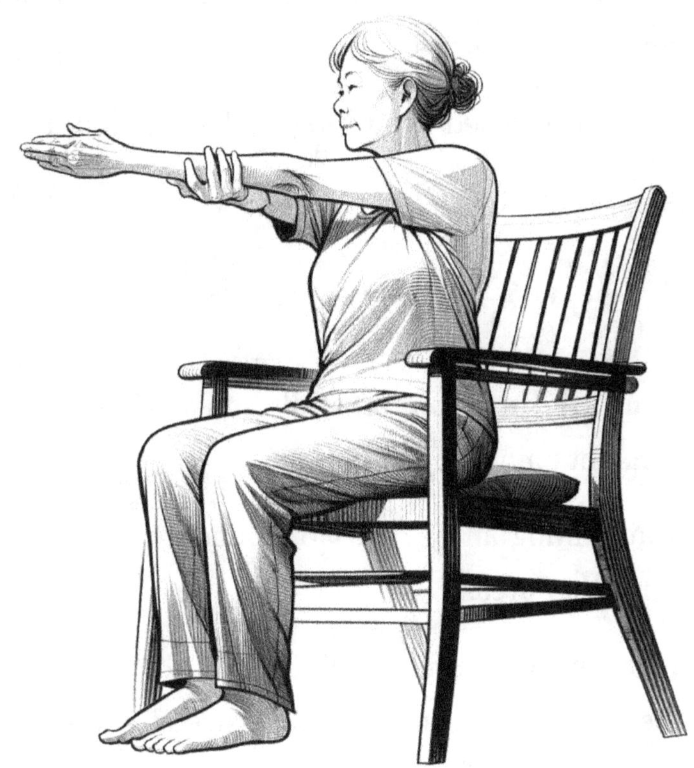

Actions

Begin in a Comfortable Seated Position: Sit in a stable chair without arms, feet flat on the floor, and maintain a straight posture.

Initiate the Stretch: Extend your right arm to the side at shoulder height, palm facing down.

Engage in the Stretch: Gently reach your right arm across your body, using your left hand to either press against your right elbow or wrap your arm further for a deeper stretch.

Hold and Breathe: Maintain the position for 3-5 deep breaths, focusing on the stretch along the outside of your shoulder.

Switch Sides: Slowly release and repeat the stretch with your left arm to ensure balance in the stretching routine.

Benefits

Reduces Shoulder Tension: Ideal for alleviating stiffness and discomfort in the shoulder region.

Increases Range of Motion: Regular practice can lead to improved flexibility and range of motion in the shoulders.

Aids in Injury Prevention: By enhancing shoulder mobility, seniors can reduce the risk of strains and injuries during daily activities.

Promotes Relaxation: The focused breathing and stretching act as a form of relaxation, reducing stress levels.

Common Mistakes

Overstretching: Extending the arm too forcefully can strain muscles. It's crucial to stretch to the point of gentle tension, not pain.

Incorrect Posture: Maintaining an upright spine ensures the stretch effectively targets the shoulder without straining other areas.

Holding Breath: Forgetting to breathe deeply during the stretch can diminish its benefits. Continuous, deep breaths enhance relaxation and the stretch's effectiveness.

Variations

Increased Stretch: For a deeper stretch, gently press the elbow with the opposite hand, encouraging the arm closer to the chest.

Reduced Intensity: If the full stretch is too intense, simply laying the arm across the body without additional pressure can offer a gentler alternative.

Standing Option: This stretch can also be performed standing, using a wall for balance if needed, catering to those who might want to incorporate standing exercises.

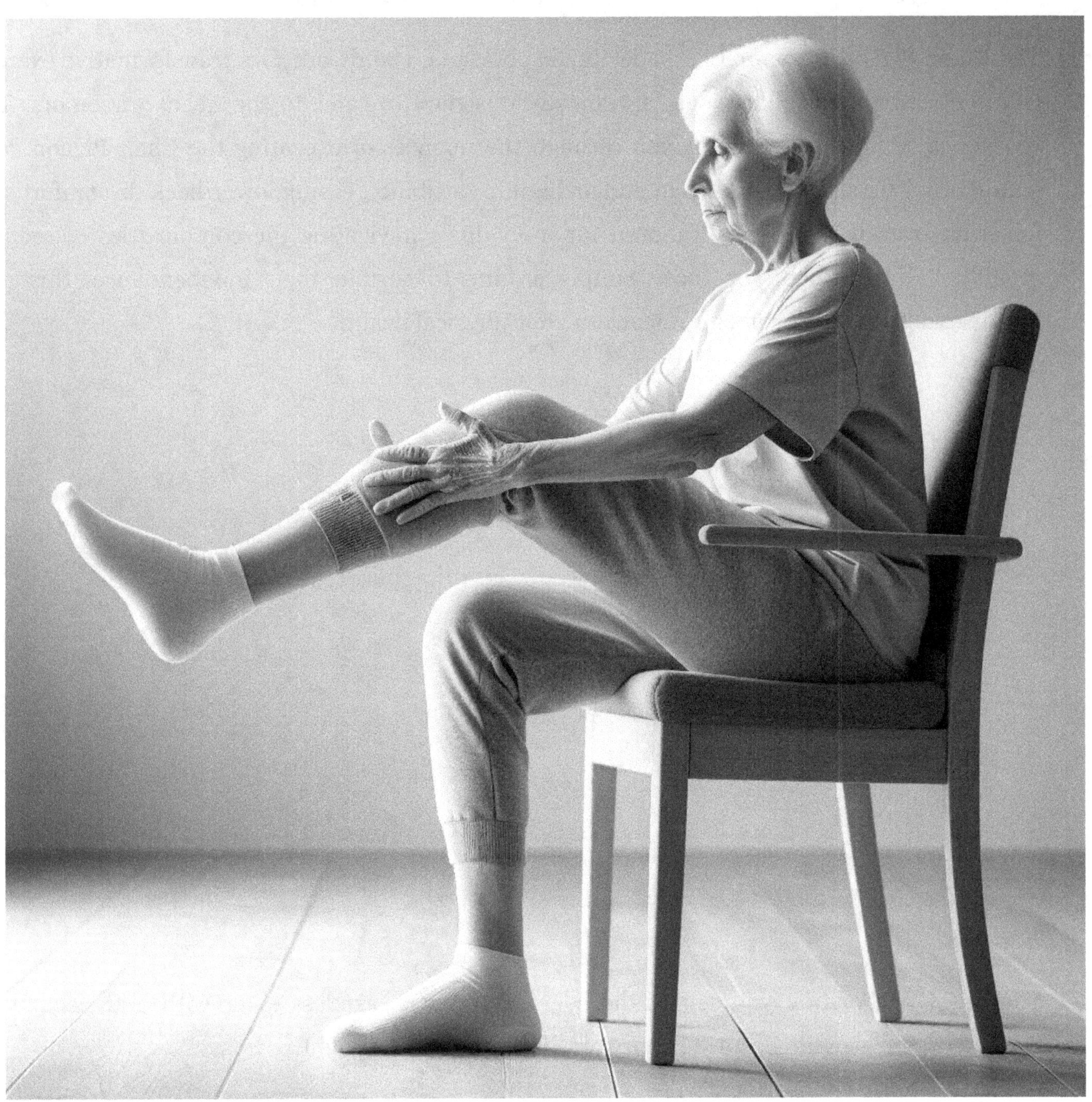

The Chair Pigeon Pose, or Eka Pada Rajakapotasana, stands out as a transformative exercise within the realm of chair yoga, specifically designed to cater to the needs of seniors. This chapter is dedicated to guiding you through the nuances of executing the Chair Pigeon Pose, highlighting its significant role in enhancing hip flexibility, easing lower back discomfort, and fostering overall well-being. Tailored for individuals navigating the complexities of reduced mobility, chronic pain, or those simply aiming to sustain their independence, this pose promises a gentle yet profound impact on your physical health.

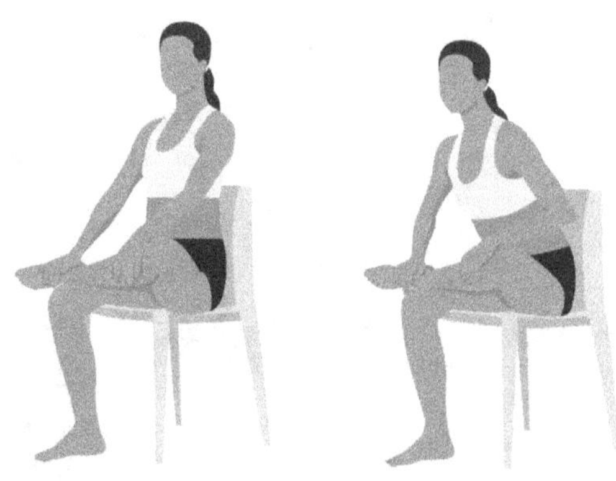

Actions

Setting Up: Position yourself at the edge of a sturdy, armless chair with both feet firmly planted on the ground, ensuring your spine is aligned and upright.

Entering the Pose: Carefully lift your right ankle, placing it atop your left thigh just above the knee, creating a figure-four shape with your legs. Keep your right knee relaxed, allowing it to gently open to the side.

Deepening the Stretch: With a straight spine, gradually lean forward from your hips, maintaining a broad chest. The depth of your lean should be guided by the stretch's comfort level in your right hip.

Releasing the Pose: After holding the pose for a few deep breaths, slowly return to an upright seated position and gently lower your right foot to the floor. Repeat the process with the left leg to ensure balance in the stretch.

Benefits

Enhanced Hip Flexibility: This pose targets the hip flexors and external rotators, helping to alleviate tightness and improve range of motion.

Lower Back Pain Relief: By stretching the muscles around the hips, the Chair Pigeon Pose can reduce strain and tension in the lower back, offering relief from discomfort.

Promotes Circulation: The positioning encourages better blood flow to the pelvic region, supporting overall hip health and function.

Common Mistakes

Overstretching: Attempting to deepen the stretch beyond your comfort level can lead to strain. Listen to your body and respect its limits.

Incorrect Posture: Slouching or rounding the back during the pose reduces its effectiveness and can cause discomfort. Ensure your spine remains straight throughout.

Forcing the Knee: Applying pressure to the knee to push it downward can lead to injury. Allow your knee to naturally lower to its comfortable range.

Variations

Supported Stretch: For additional support, place a cushion or yoga block under the raised knee to help relax into the pose without strain.

Increased Intensity: For a deeper stretch, once in the pose and maintaining proper alignment, gently press down on the raised knee with your hand, increasing the stretch in the outer hip.

Alternative Leg Position: If placing your ankle on the opposite thigh is too challenging, simply cross your ankles, keeping both feet on the ground, and lean forward to feel a gentler stretch in the hips.

The Seated Spinal Twist, or Ardha Matsyendrasana in a chair, is a fundamental chair yoga pose designed to enhance spinal mobility, improve digestion, and relieve back pain. This chapter guides seniors through safely executing the Seated Spinal Twist, highlighting its benefits, common mistakes to avoid, and variations to accommodate different mobility levels.

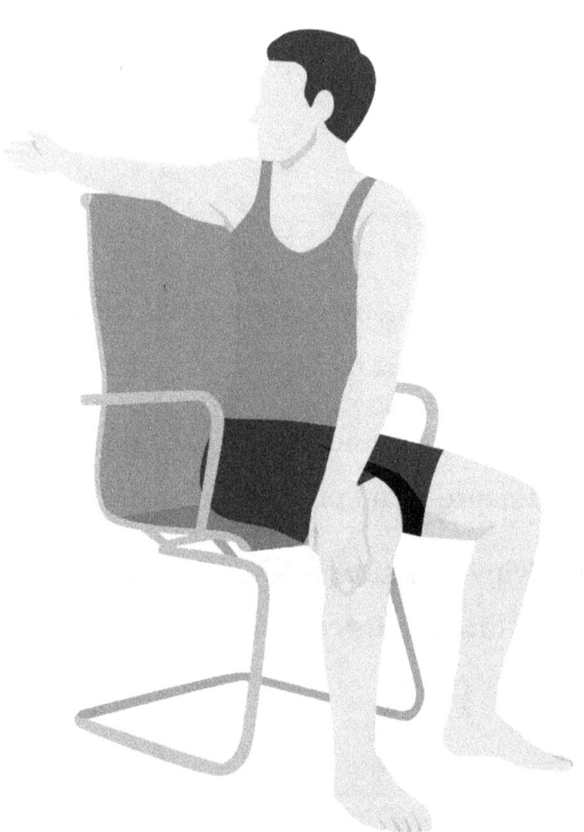

Actions

Start with the Right Setup: Sit squarely in your chair, feet flat on the ground, hips width apart. Ensure your back is straight, and your shoulders are relaxed.

Engage in the Twist: Place your right hand on the back of the chair. Use your left hand on the outside of your right knee as leverage to gently twist your torso to the right. Keep your chin aligned with your shoulder to ensure the twist involves the spine uniformly, from the base to the neck.

Repeat on the Other Side: Return to the center and repeat the twist on the opposite side to maintain balance in flexibility and strength throughout your spine.

Benefits

Enhanced Spinal Mobility: Regular practice of this twist can increase the flexibility and range of motion in the spine, contributing to improved posture.

Stimulation of Digestion: The twisting motion massages internal organs, helping to stimulate digestion and detoxification.

Reduction of Back Pain: By stretching and strengthening the muscles around the spine, this pose can contribute to reduced back pain.

Common Mistakes

Over-Twisting: Avoid forcing the twist, which can strain the back. The motion should be gentle and controlled.

Holding the Breath: Breathing should be steady and deep. Holding your breath can create tension in the body, counteracting the pose's benefits.

Misalignment: Keep your hips square and avoid leaning forward or back. Misalignment can reduce the effectiveness of the twist and risk discomfort or injury.

Variations

For Increased Challenge: To deepen the twist, look over your shoulder in the direction of the twist, but only if it feels comfortable for your neck.

For Gentle Practice: If the twist feels too intense, simply place your hands on your lap and use your core muscles to initiate the twist without leveraging your arms.

Core Engagement and Stability

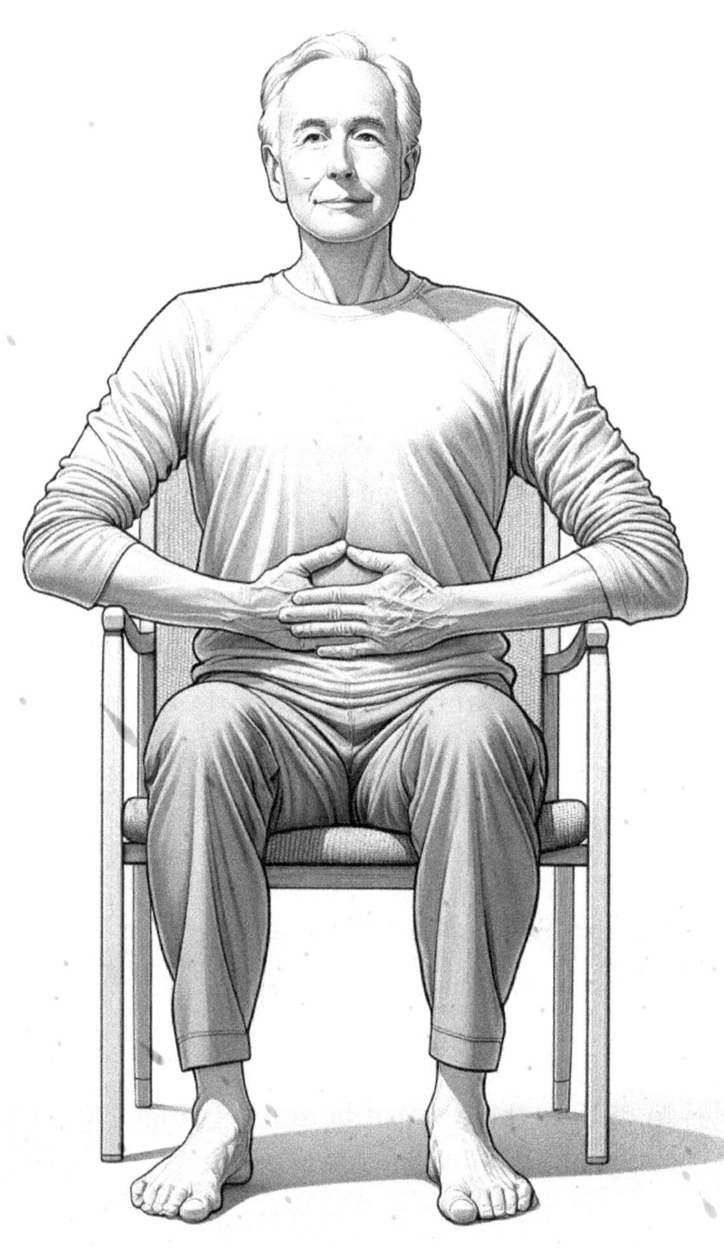

The Seated Mountain Pose, or Tadasana in a seated form, serves as the cornerstone of chair yoga, offering a unique blend of simplicity and profound impact. This fundamental pose is designed to ground seniors, fostering a sense of stability and presence. It is the starting point from which all other chair yoga poses can unfold, providing a foundation for both physical and mental well-being.

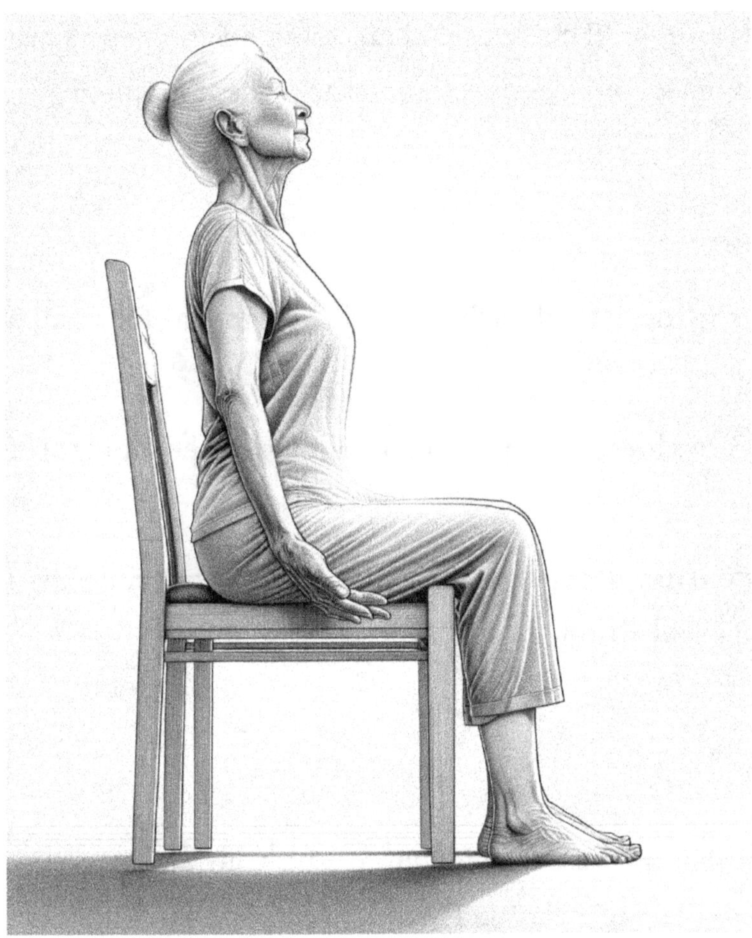

Actions

Finding Your Seat: Begin by sitting at the edge of a sturdy, armless chair with your feet planted firmly on the ground. This position encourages proper alignment and prepares your body for the pose.

Elevating the Spine: With a deep inhale, imagine a string pulling your head towards the ceiling, elongating your spine. Keep your shoulders relaxed and your gaze forward, embodying the majesty of a mountain.

Engaging Your Core: Gently engage your abdominal muscles, drawing your navel towards your spine. This subtle engagement is crucial for stability and supports the integrity of the pose.

Benefits

Improved Posture: Regular practice of the Seated Mountain Pose encourages alignment of the spine, shoulders, and head, combating the tendency to slouch and mitigating back pain.

Enhanced Breathing: The upright posture opens up the chest, allowing for deeper, more efficient breathing, which is vital for overall health and stress reduction.

Increased Awareness: This pose fosters a heightened sense of bodily awareness, encouraging mindfulness and a connection to the present moment.

Common Mistakes:

Overarching the Spine: Avoid pushing your chest too far forward, which can strain the back. Aim for a natural, straight alignment.

Tightening the Shoulders: Keep your shoulders relaxed and away from your ears to prevent tension buildup.

Forgetting to Breathe: It's easy to hold your breath while focusing on posture. Remember to breathe deeply and evenly throughout the pose.

Variations

Arm Extensions: For added engagement, extend your arms overhead, keeping them parallel to each other, palms facing inward. This variation enhances the stretch along the spine and engages the upper body.

Foot Lifts: Alternately lift your feet a few inches off the ground, maintaining balance and stability. This variation adds a gentle challenge to your leg muscles and core.

The Seated Forward Bend, or Paschimottanasana adapted for chair yoga, is a gentle, accessible exercise that brings profound benefits, particularly for seniors. This chapter delves into the nuances of performing the Seated Forward Bend with safety and effectiveness in mind, highlighting its significance in enhancing flexibility, relieving stress, and promoting a deep sense of relaxation.

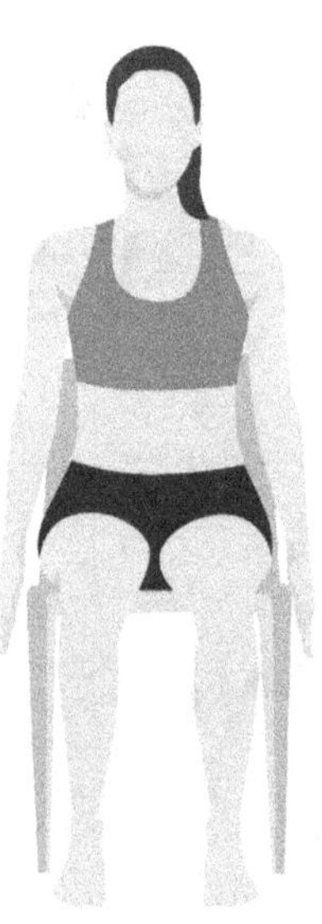
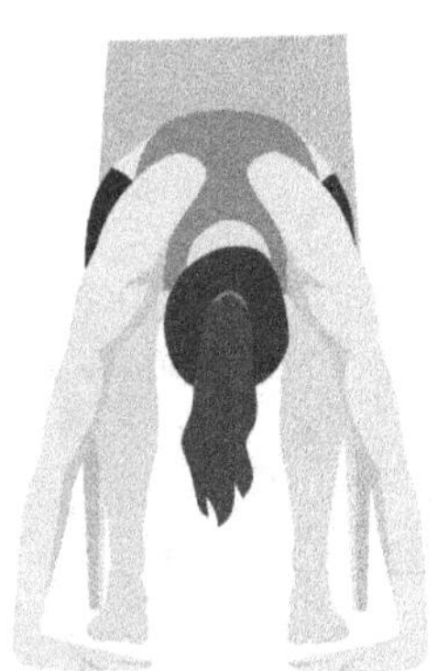

Actions

Finding Your Seat: Choosing the right chair is crucial. It should provide a stable base without being too soft. Your feet should rest firmly on the ground, creating a 90-degree angle at your knees, which aligns your posture before you begin.

Initiate the Movement: Starting with a deep inhalation, visualize lengthening your spine as though a string is pulling you upwards from the crown of your head. This upward extension is vital for preparing your body for the forward motion.

Deepen the Stretch: As you exhale and fold forward, lead with your chest to maintain a flat back, aiming to bring your abdomen closer to your thighs. This mindful progression ensures you're stretching correctly without compromising your form.

Benefits

Encourages spinal flexibility and stretches the lower back: Regularly practicing this pose can significantly reduce stiffness and discomfort in your back, promoting a more supple and flexible spine, essential for daily activities.

Stimulates abdominal organs, aiding in digestion: The forward bending motion massages internal organs, particularly the digestive system, which can improve metabolism and alleviate digestion-related issues.

Calms the mind, reducing symptoms of stress and mild anxiety: The focused breathing and gentle forward fold act as a physical metaphor for letting go of stress, encouraging a peaceful state of mind.

Common Mistakes

Rounding the Back: This common error can lead to strain. Imagine lengthening your torso with each inhale and deepening your fold with each exhale to maintain the integrity of the stretch.

Forcing the Stretch: Honoring your body's limits is key. Flexibility will increase over time, so there's no need to push yourself to the point of discomfort.

Neglecting Breathing: The breath is your guide through the stretch. Coordinate your movements with your inhales and exhales to deepen the effectiveness of the pose and maintain focus.

Variations

With Support: Using a cushion or yoga block not only provides support but also helps maintain proper alignment and deepen the stretch safely, making the pose accessible regardless of flexibility level.

Arm Variation: Raising the arms overhead introduces an additional element of balance and stretches the sides of the body. This variation can intensify the stretch along the spine and shoulders, increasing the pose's benefits.

Chapter 6:

Chair Yoga Poses for Flexibility

Gentle Stretches for Improved Mobility

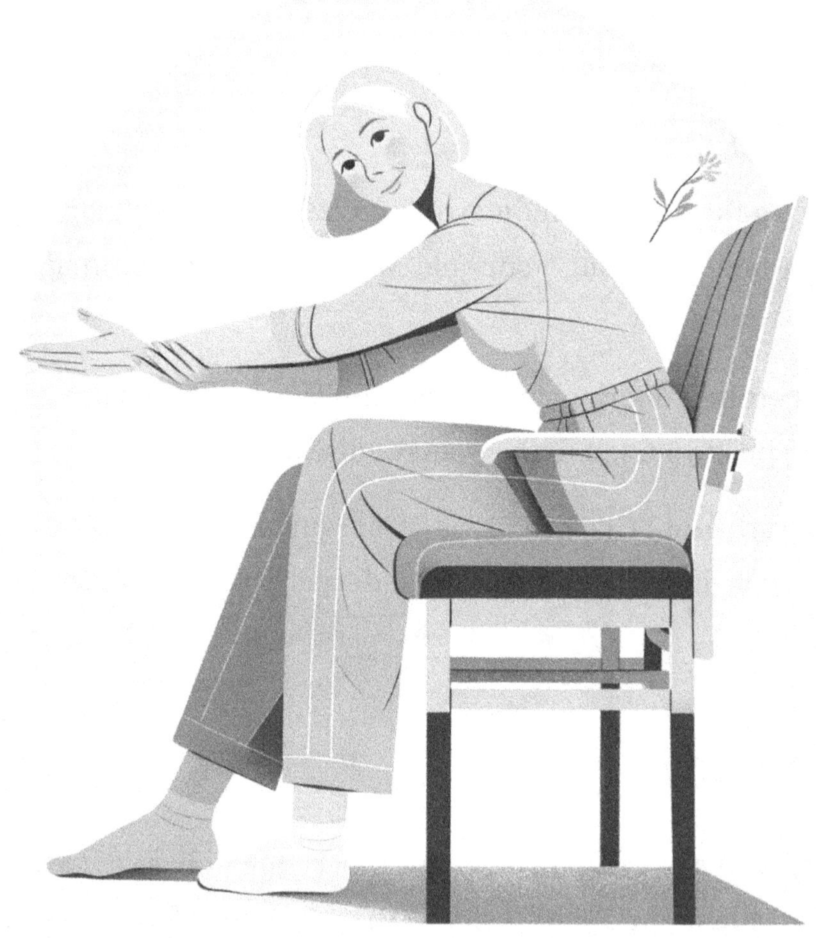

In the journey toward holistic well-being, particularly for seniors, the significance of nurturing neck health cannot be overstated. The Neck Rolls presents a gentle yet powerful chair yoga exercise designed to alleviate the stiffness and discomfort that often accumulates in the neck region. This chapter is dedicated to guiding you through the simple, yet transformative, practice of neck rolls, a cornerstone exercise in chair yoga that targets the delicate structures of the neck. Through careful, mindful movement, neck rolls offer a pathway to not only easing tension but also to enhancing overall mobility and quality of life. Whether you're navigating the challenges of reduced mobility, seeking relief from chronic pain, or simply striving to maintain independence and vitality in your later years, this exercise stands as a testament to the gentle power of chair yoga. Let's embark on this journey together, exploring step-by-step instructions, key benefits, and thoughtful variations to tailor this practice to your unique needs and enhance your chair yoga experience.

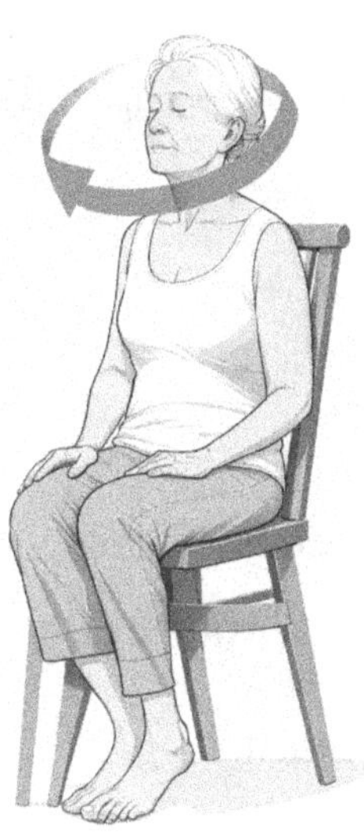

Actions

Finding Your Seat: Start by sitting comfortably in a sturdy chair, feet grounded and spine straight.

Initiate Neck Rolls: Gently lower your chin to your chest to start the circular motion.

Roll Your Neck Slowly: Move your head to the right, bringing your ear towards the shoulder, then gently roll your head back and then to the left side, completing the circle by bringing your chin back to your chest.

Repeat: Continue the movement for a few cycles, then change direction.

Benefits

Relieves Neck Tension: Regular practice can significantly reduce stiffness and discomfort.

Improves Flexibility: Increases the range of motion in the neck, aiding in everyday activities.

Reduces Stress: The rhythmic movement can have a calming effect, lowering stress levels.

Common Mistakes

Moving Too Quickly: Rapid movements can strain the neck. Emphasize the importance of slow, deliberate motions.

Forcing the Motion: Advise against pushing the neck beyond its comfortable range of motion to prevent injury.

Ignoring Pain: Encourage readers to stop immediately if they experience pain, emphasizing the gentle nature of the exercise.

Variations

Partial Rolls: For those with severe stiffness, recommend limiting the movement to a semi-circle, moving from one shoulder to the chin and then to the other shoulder.

Assisted Stretch: Suggest using a hand to gently guide the head in the roll, adding a slight manual stretch to enhance the exercise's benefits.

This chapter unveils the simplicity and profound impact of extending one's body skyward. This fundamental yet powerful pose serves as a cornerstone for enhancing flexibility, relieving tension, and fostering a deep sense of rejuvenation. Tailored for seniors seeking to maintain or reclaim their mobility and independence, this guide offers a pathway to improved posture and vitality. Through careful instruction and mindful practice, the Overhead Stretch becomes more than a physical exercise; it transforms into a ritual of reaching towards one's fullest potential.

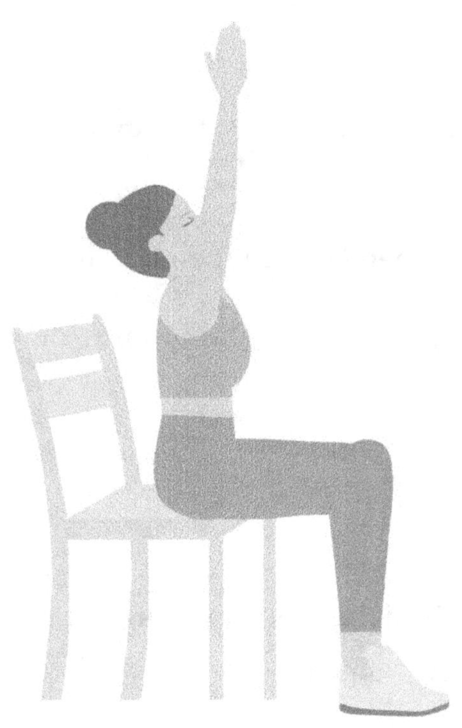

Actions

Finding Your Seat: Encourage sitting in a sturdy, armless chair, feet planted firmly on the ground, spine erect.

Initiate the Stretch: Instruct to inhale deeply while raising both arms overhead, palms facing each other.

Deepen the Stretch: Suggest reaching higher with each exhale, stretching the spine and ribcage upward.

Hold and Release: Advise holding the stretch for a few breaths, then slowly lowering the arms on an exhale.

Benefits

Improves Posture: Helps realign the spine and shoulders, promoting a more upright posture.

Increases Flexibility: Stretches the arms, shoulders, and upper back, enhancing flexibility.

Boosts Circulation: Elevating the arms overhead can improve blood flow to the upper body and brain.

Common Mistakes

Straining the Neck: Warn against lifting the shoulders too high, which can compress the neck.

Locking the Elbows: Recommend a slight bend in the elbows to prevent hyperextension.

Holding the Breath: Emphasize the importance of continuous breathing to maximize benefits.

Variations

With a Strap: For those with tight shoulders, suggest holding a yoga strap or towel between the hands to keep them properly aligned.

One Arm at a Time: Offer an option to stretch one arm overhead at a time, which can be more comfortable for some.

The Seated Side Stretch is a quintessential exercise in chair yoga, designed to promote flexibility, alleviate stiffness, and enhance mobility in the upper and lower back. Ideal for seniors, this exercise encourages gentle stretching of the spine through side bending, providing relief and contributing to overall spinal health. This chapter will guide you through the steps, benefits, common mistakes, and variations of the Seated Side Stretch, ensuring a comprehensive understanding and effective practice.

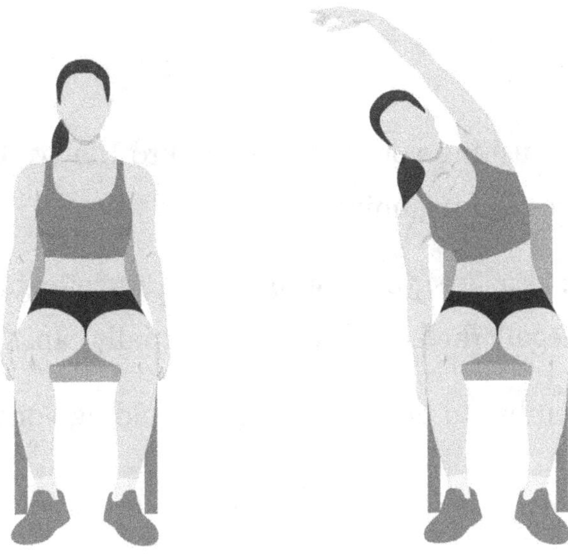

Actions

Finding Your Seat: Begin by sitting comfortably in an armless chair, feet flat on the floor, and spine in a neutral, upright position.

Initiating the Stretch: Place one hand on the side of the chair for support. Inhale deeply, and as you exhale, gently slide your other hand down the corresponding leg of the chair, bending your spine sideways.

Increasing the Stretch: To intensify the stretch, raise the opposite arm above your head, creating additional leverage. Ensure your movement is controlled and smooth.

Repeating on the Other Side: Gradually return to the starting position, and repeat the stretch on the opposite side for balanced flexibility.

Benefits

Spinal Mobility: This exercise significantly improves the range of motion in your spine, combating the stiffness that comes with age.

Upper and Lower Back Relief: Regular practice helps relieve tension and discomfort in both the upper and lower back regions.

Improved Posture: By enhancing spinal flexibility, the Seated Side Stretch contributes to better posture, reducing the risk of back pain.

Common Mistakes

Overstretching: Avoid pushing yourself too far into the stretch, which could lead to strain. Listen to your body and respect its limits.

Rounding the Back: Ensure your spine remains elongated throughout the exercise. Rounding the back can negate the benefits and potentially cause discomfort.

Holding Breath: Remember to breathe steadily. Holding your breath can create unnecessary tension in your body.

Variations

Arm Position Adjustment: For those with shoulder issues, keep both hands on your lap and focus solely on the side bending of the spine.

Added Support: Place a cushion or folded towel on your lap, and gently rest your elbow on it as you bend to the side, reducing the intensity for beginners or those with severe stiffness.

Dynamic Movement: Incorporate a gentle, rhythmic motion by alternating sides in a flowing manner, enhancing the mobilization of the spine.

Embrace the strength and courage of a warrior with Chair Warrior I, a pose that brings the traditional Virabhadrasana I to your chair. This adaptation is not just about maintaining balance and strength; it's a celebration of your capacity for resilience and independence. This chapter guides you through mastering Chair Warrior I, designed for seniors aiming to enhance mobility, strength, and maintain their independence, despite challenges like reduced mobility or chronic pain.

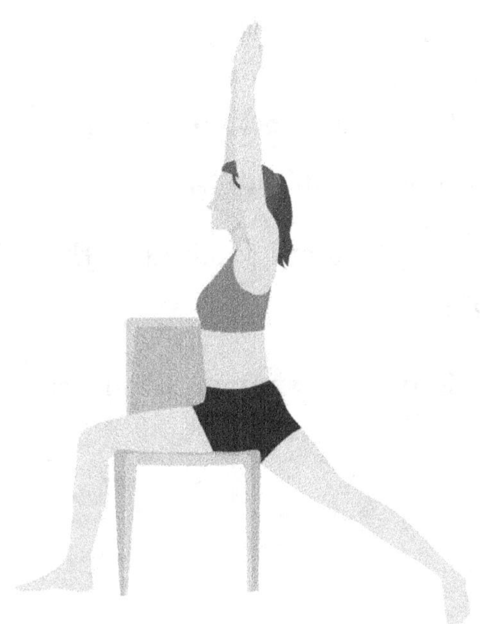

Actions

Positioning Your Chair: Start by placing your chair sideways so that you can sit comfortably with one leg on each side, ensuring it's stable and won't move.

Establishing Your Base: Sit on the chair sideways with your right thigh over the side. Extend your left leg straight back, keeping both feet flat and grounded to maintain stability.

Raising Into Strength: Inhale and lift your arms overhead, bringing your palms to face each other, stretching through your fingertips as if reaching towards the sky.

Engaging Your Core: As you exhale, gently turn your torso towards your right leg, ensuring your hips remain squared to the front, engaging your core for balance and stability.

Switching Sides: Hold the pose for a few breaths, then gently release and switch sides to ensure balance in your practice.

Benefits

Enhances lower body strength, particularly in the legs and hips.

Improves focus and concentration through balanced posture.

Increases spinal flexibility and encourages a gentle stretch in the torso.

Stimulates abdominal organs, aiding in digestion and overall well-being.

Common Mistakes

Overstraining the Neck: Keep your neck in line with your spine to avoid strain. Your gaze should be forward or slightly upward, not tilting back.

Misaligned Hips: Ensure your hips are squared to the front of the room, not tilting to one side, to maintain proper alignment.

Forgetting to Breathe: Maintain a smooth, even breath throughout the pose to support movement and stability.

Variations

Arm Variations: For those with shoulder issues, instead of raising arms overhead, place hands on the hips or the back of the chair for support.

Leg Position: If extending the back leg straight causes discomfort, keep both feet on the ground and focus on the torso and arm movement.

Intensity Adjustment: To increase the challenge, deepen the bend in your seated leg or hold the pose longer, focusing on deep, steady breaths.

Chair Yoga Poses for Balance

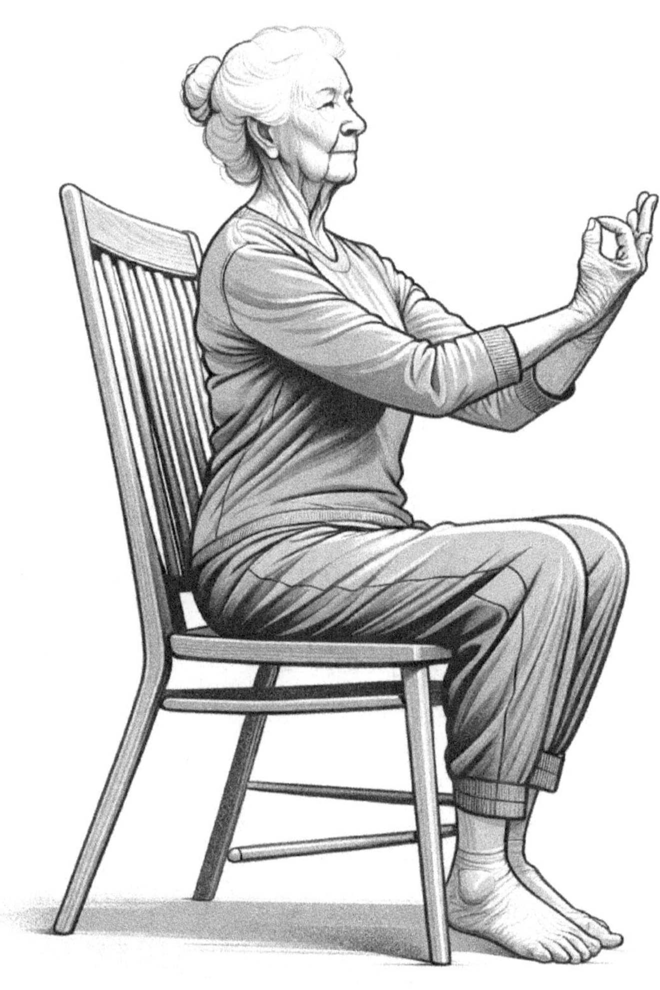

As we continue our journey through chair yoga, let's explore the Seated Eagle Pose (Garudasana). This graceful and empowering posture offers a unique blend of strength, flexibility, and mental focus. Whether you're a seasoned practitioner or a curious beginner, Seated Eagle Pose invites you to ride the winds of transformation and discover newfound stability.

In this chapter, we'll break down the Seated Eagle Pose step by step, emphasizing alignment, modifications, and the profound benefits it brings. As we delve into this pose, remember that it's not just about physical movement; it's about connecting with your inner resilience and embracing the freedom to soar.

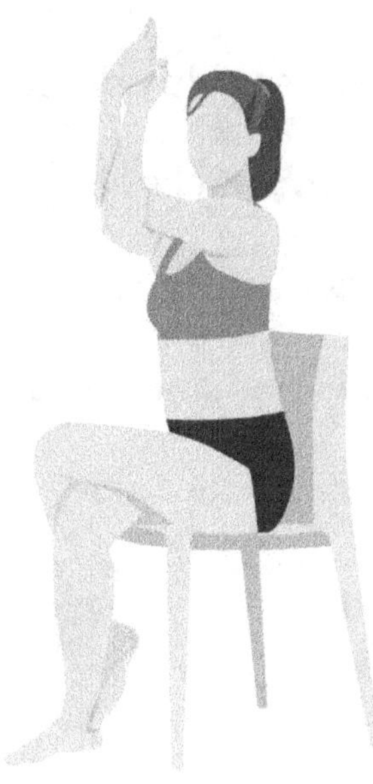

Finding Your Seat: Begin with Steadiness

Before we dive into the intricacies of Seated Eagle Pose, let's find our foundation:

Sukhasana (Easy Pose):

- Sit comfortably on your chair, spine erect, and feet grounded.
- Cross your legs, allowing your knees to fall gently outward.
- Rest your hands on your thighs, palms facing down.
- Breathe deeply, settling into the present moment.

Actions

Eagle Arms:

- Extend your arms forward at shoulder height.
- Cross your right arm over your left, bringing your palms to touch.
- Bend your elbows, allowing your forearms to wrap around each other.
- Lift your elbows slightly, creating a gentle resistance.
- Keep your shoulders relaxed and your gaze steady.

Leg Variation: Cross your right leg over your left, if comfortable. If balance is a concern, keep your right foot grounded or use a block for support.Feel the engagement in your thighs and ankles.

Benefits

Balance and Focus: Seated Eagle Pose cultivates mental clarity and concentration.

Shoulder and Upper Back Stretch: It releases tension in the shoulders and upper back.

Core Strength: The crossed arms activate the core muscles.

Improved Posture: Regular practice enhances spinal alignment.

Stress Relief: The focused breath calms the mind.

Common Mistakes

Over-Twisting: Avoid excessive twisting; maintain a comfortable range of motion.

Tension in Shoulders: Keep your shoulders away from your ears.

Neglecting the Legs: Engage both legs equally for stability.

Variations

Seated Eagle Pose with Kickstand: Cross your legs without wrapping your feet completely. Place your foot on the ground or a block for balance.

Eagle Pose in a Chair: Practice the pose while seated in a chair. Focus on the upper body alignment without worrying about balance.

As we traverse the golden years, our journey towards maintaining health and vitality becomes ever more poignant. Spinal health is the crux of our mobility and independence, and the Chair Warrior II pose, or as we'll refer to it, the Seated Spinal Twist, is a beacon on this path. This chapter delves into the empowering practice of the Seated Spinal Twist, guiding you to enhance your strength and vitality from the comfort of your chair.

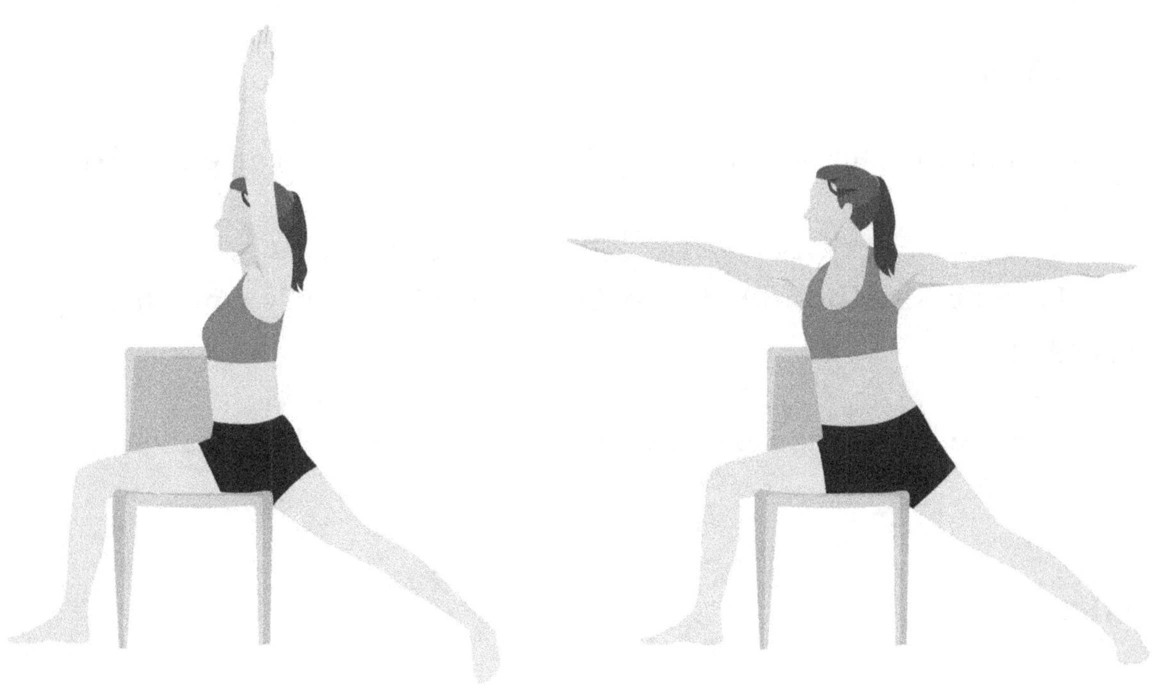

Actions

Finding Your Seat: Begin by sitting on the chair sideways, ensuring that both sit bones are evenly supported. Feel grounded through your seat.

Positioning Your Legs: Extend your leading leg to the side, planting your foot firmly. Stretch the other leg back, foot perpendicular, feeling the stability from the hips.

Embracing the Horizon: Spread your arms parallel to the ground, radiate energy through your fingertips, and gaze past the front hand, embodying the warrior within.

Balancing Your Practice: Hold the pose, breathe deeply, and on each exhale, sink a little deeper into the strength of your legs. Switch sides to maintain balance.

Benefits

Leg Strength: This pose fortifies leg muscles, crucial for daily activities.

Stability and Balance: Enhances core strength, reducing the risk of falls.

Hip and Chest Opening: Encourages flexibility and relieves tightness in the chest and hips.

Common Mistakes

Overreaching: Extending too far can strain muscles. Ensure alignment and comfort in every pose.

Uneven Weight Distribution: Both sit bones should be equally supported to prevent spinal misalignment.

Holding Breath: Breathing should be steady and deep, not held or shallow.

Variations

For Added Support: Use a cushion for comfort or a block under the extended leg's foot if it doesn't reach the ground.

Intensity Modification: For a gentler pose, keep the back leg slightly bent. For more intensity, actively engage the thigh muscles of the extended legs.

As we embrace the autumn of our lives, it's vital to nourish the roots of our well-being. The Chair Tree Pose, or Vrksasana, is a testament to the enduring strength and balance we can cultivate through chair yoga. This pose allows us to ground ourselves in the present, fostering stability and clarity in both body and mind.

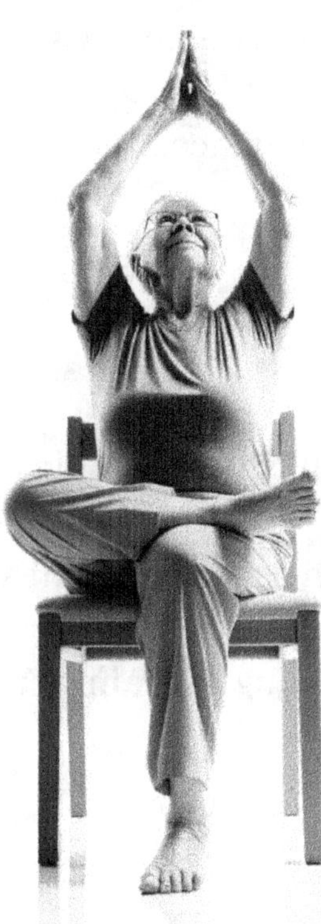

Actions

Finding Your Seat: Begin by sitting firmly on the chair, feet flat on the ground, spine tall and dignified. Engage your core gently to support your upright posture.

Planting the Seed: Place the sole of your right foot against the inner thigh or calf of your left leg. Avoid placing it on the knee to prevent strain. Press your foot and thigh together, creating a mutual support system.

Growing Your Branches: Bring your palms together in Anjali Mudra (prayer position) at your heart center, or raise your arms overhead like the branches of a tree, keeping your shoulders soft and face relaxed. Find a drishti, or focal point, that's unmoving to aid your balance.

Repeating the Cycle: Hold the pose for 5-10 breaths, feeling the steadiness of your seated trunk. Gently release and repeat on the other side, ensuring balance in practice.

Benefits:

Improves focus and concentration.

Strengthens the ankles, thighs, and core muscles while seated.

Encourages thoracic (upper back) spine mobility when arms are raised.

Cultivates a sense of grounding and balance.

Common Mistakes:

Rushing into the pose without establishing a stable base.

Placing the foot on the knee, which can cause joint strain.

Holding breath—keep the breath flowing to maintain balance and focus.

Variations:

For those with hip restrictions, place the foot lower on the calf or ankle.

Arms can remain on the hips if raising them causes shoulder discomfort.

For an extra challenge, try closing your eyes for a breath or two.

Chapter 8

Chair Yoga Poses for Knee and Back Pain

The gentle practice of Chair Yoga is a beacon of hope for those seeking relief from knee pain and back discomfort. As we age, our joints may begin to stiffen and our spines can lose flexibility, leading to aches and limitations in movement. The beauty of Chair Yoga lies in its ability to provide a safe and supportive environment for seniors to nurture their bodies with mindful movement.

For those grappling with knee issues, the Chair Yoga practice offers a sanctuary of healing. The seated postures allow for a gradual opening of the hips and knees, promoting increased circulation and lubrication within the joints. By gently stretching and strengthening the muscles surrounding the knees, Chair Yoga helps to improve stability and reduce the impact of daily activities on this vital joint. Through consistent practice, many seniors find that their knee discomfort lessens, granting them the freedom to move with greater ease and comfort.

Knee Health

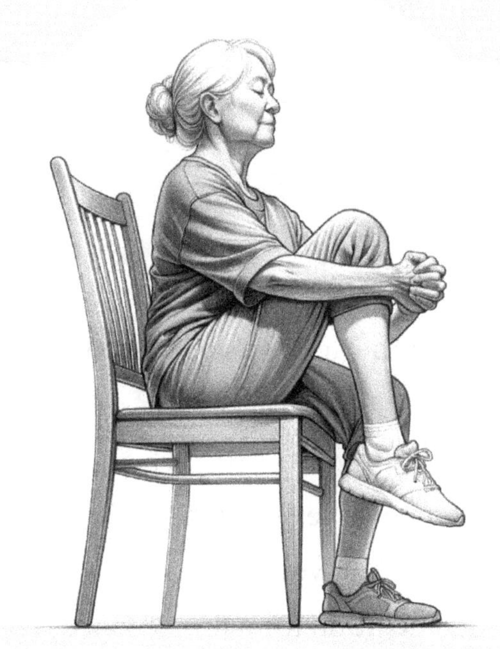

Let us embark on a journey that celebrates the resilience of your legs—the **Seated Leg Extensions**. Imagine sitting tall, your feet grounded, and your spirit soaring. In this pose, we honor the very foundation that supports your independence. Whether you seek to regain strength or simply revel in the joy of movement, this chapter is your sanctuary.

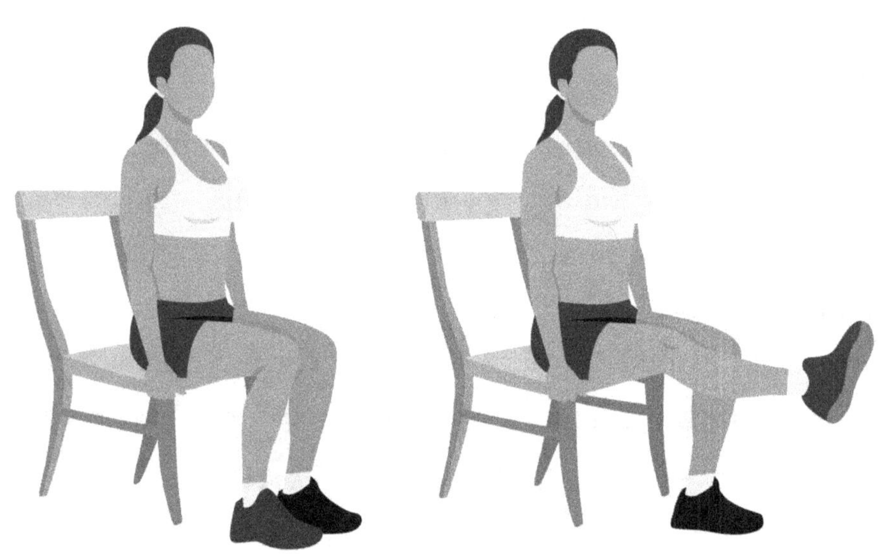

Actions: Elevating Your Legs

1. **Finding Your Seat**:
   - Sit comfortably on a sturdy chair, spine erect, and feet flat on the floor.
   - Place your hands on the armrests or your thighs for support.
2. **Leg Extension Flow**:
   - Inhale deeply, engaging your core.
   - Exhale as you extend one leg straight out in front of you.
   - Keep your toes flexed and your knee soft (avoid locking it).
   - Hold the extended position for a few seconds, feeling the stretch in your quadriceps.
3. **Return Gracefully**:
   - Inhale again, and with control, lower your leg back down.
   - Alternate between legs, maintaining a steady rhythm.

Benefits: Fortifying Your Foundation

- **Quadriceps Activation**: Seated Leg Extensions target the quadriceps—the mighty muscles at the front of your thighs. These powerhouses help you rise from chairs, climb stairs, and walk confidently.
- **Knee Stability**: By strengthening the quadriceps, you enhance knee stability, reducing the risk of falls and supporting joint health.
- **Improved Circulation**: Elevating your legs encourages blood flow, reducing swelling and promoting overall vitality.
- **Functional Independence**: Imagine effortlessly reaching for a high shelf or stepping onto a bus. Seated Leg Extensions empower these everyday movements.

Common Mistakes: Treading Lightly

- **Overextension**: Avoid locking your knee. Keep a gentle bend to protect your joint.
- **Speedy Movements**: Slow and deliberate wins the race. Rushing compromises form and effectiveness.
- **Neglecting Breath**: Breathe mindfully. Inhale during extension, exhale during lowering.

Variations: Tailoring the Experience

1. **Ankle Weights Adventure**:
    - Strap on ankle weights (start with 5 pounds and progress to 10 pounds).
    - Extend your legs, feeling the added resistance.
    - Imagine your quads growing stronger with each lift.
2. **Resistance Band Delight**:
    - Loop a resistance band around your ankles.
    - Sit tall and extend your legs against the band's tension.
    - Feel the burn as you engage your quads.

Imagine your ankles as the silent guardians of your mobility—the hinges that allow you to step into life's adventures. In this chapter, we unravel the magic of **Ankle Circles**, a simple yet profound practice that honors these unsung heroes. Whether you've danced through decades or are just beginning your journey, let's embrace ankle health with reverence.

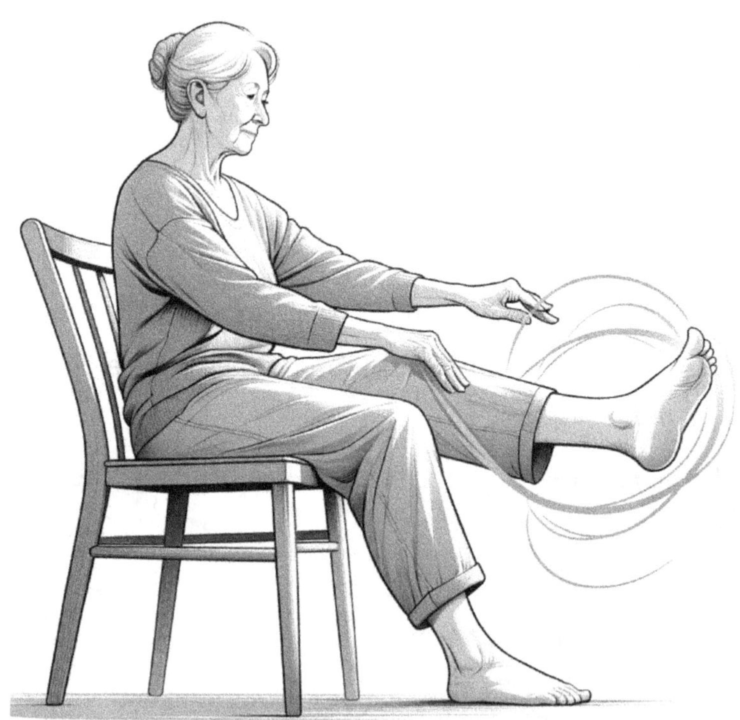

Actions: Nurturing Your Ankles

1. **Finding Your Seat**:
   - Sit comfortably on a chair, spine tall, and feet flat on the floor.
   - Place your hands on your thighs or hold the sides of the chair for stability.
2. **Circle with Grace**:
   - Lift your right foot slightly off the ground.
   - Begin rotating your right ankle in gentle circles.
   - Imagine drawing a halo with your toes—clockwise and then counterclockwise.
   - Feel the fluidity in your ankle joint.
3. **Switch Sides**:
   - Lower your right foot and repeat the same circles with your left ankle.
   - Breathe deeply, allowing the movement to flow.

Benefits: Ankle Alchemy

- **Joint Mobility**: Ankle circles lubricate the ankle joint, enhancing its range of motion. Picture your ankles as well-oiled gears, ready for any twist life throws your way.
- **Stress Relief**: As you trace those circles, tension melts away. Ankles carry the weight of your world; let them release and rejuvenate.
- **Improved Balance**: Strong, flexible ankles are your allies in maintaining balance. Whether you're navigating uneven terrain or dancing in your living room, ankle circles fortify stability.

Common Mistakes: Treading Lightly

- **Forceful Circles**: Remember, this isn't a race. Gentle rotations suffice. Avoid straining your ankles.
- **Neglecting Both Directions**: Explore clockwise and counterclockwise circles. Balance the energy flow in both directions.

Variations: Tailoring the Flow

1. **Seated Ankle Alphabet**:
   - Imagine your big toe as a pen.
   - Write the alphabet in the air using ankle movements.
   - From A to Z, explore the full range of ankle flexion.
2. **Standing Ankle Circles**:
   - Stand near a sturdy surface for support.
   - Lift one foot off the ground.
   - Circle your ankle while maintaining balance.
   - Switch to the other foot.

Back Pain

Similarly, for individuals battling persistent back pain, the Chair Yoga practice serves as a ray of light in the darkness of discomfort.

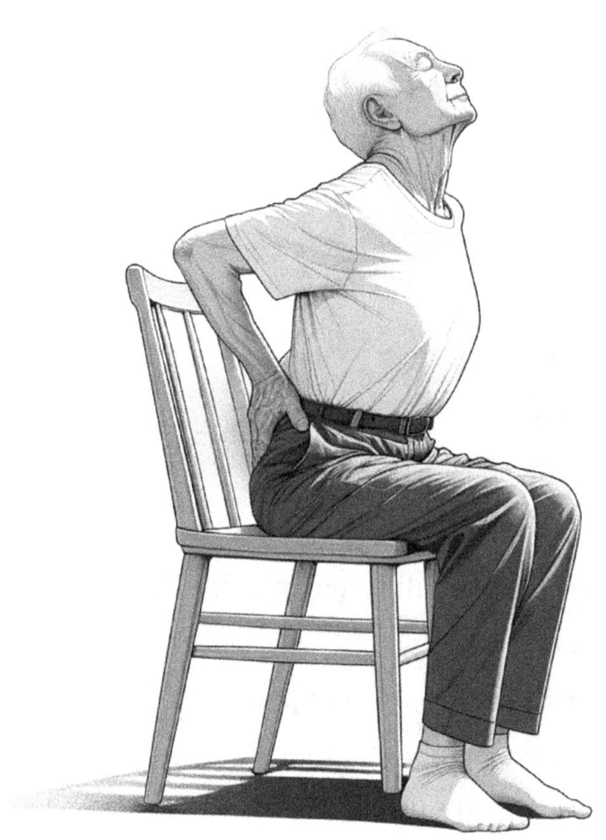

Embrace the gentle power of chair yoga with the Seated Extended Side Angle Pose—a movement that invites openness and expansion into your daily life. This pose is a celebration of your body's ability to stretch and strengthen, regardless of age. Let's explore this pose step by step, uncover its many benefits, and ensure you can practice it safely and effectively.

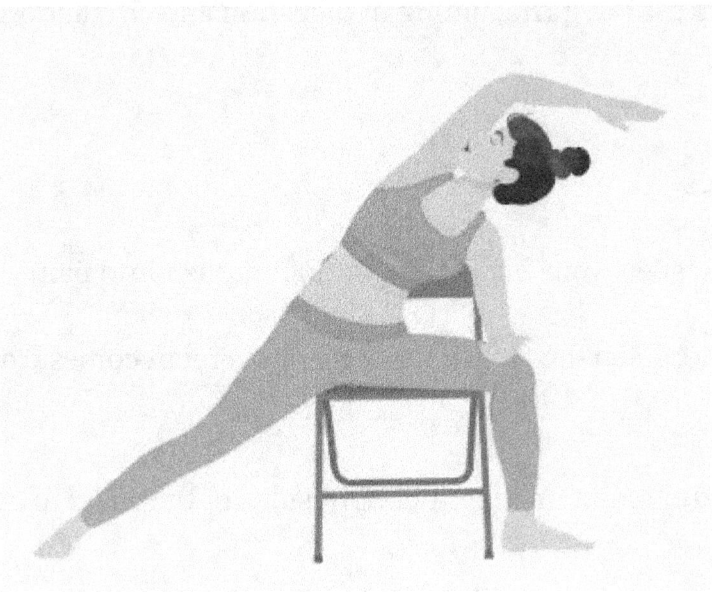

Actions

Finding Your Seat: Begin by sitting comfortably in your chair, feet flat on the floor, spine long.

Positioning Your Legs: Extend your right leg out to the side, toes pointing forward, and keep your left foot grounded.

Setting Your Base: Place your left hand on your left thigh, ensuring your seat is stable.

Reaching Up: Stretch your right arm overhead, palm facing down, and lean gently towards the left side without collapsing the waist.

Opening the Chest: Rotate your torso slightly, opening up the chest towards the ceiling, keeping your gaze upwards.

Holding the Pose: Maintain the pose for three to five deep breaths, focusing on the stretch along your right side.

Switching Sides: Gently come back to the center and repeat on the opposite side for balance.

Benefits

Enhances flexibility in the spine, shoulders, and pelvic region.

Relieves tension and discomfort in the lower back.

Encourages deep breathing, which promotes relaxation and stress relief.

Stimulates abdominal organs, aiding in digestion and circulation.

Common Mistakes

Overstretching: Respect your body's limits; do not push into pain.

Twisting the Spine: Keep the twist gentle; the movement comes from the side bend, not the twist.

Collapsing the Side: Maintain length in both sides of the waist to avoid compressing the lower side.

Losing the Seat: Ensure both sitting bones remain in contact with the chair for stability.

Variations

With Support: Place a yoga block or cushion under your extended hand for support if reaching the floor is uncomfortable.

For More Stability: Keep both feet on the ground and simply lean to the side with the arm extended, if extending the leg out is too challenging.

Increase the Stretch: For a deeper stretch, tilt your head to look past your extended arm.

In this chapter, we explore the **Chair Sphinx Pose**, a gentle yet transformative backbend that nourishes your spine and opens your heart. As you embark on this journey, envision the ancient wisdom of the Sphinx guiding you toward greater well-being.

The Sphinx, a mythical creature with the body of a lion and the head of a human, symbolizes strength, wisdom, and guardianship. In our chair adaptation, we invoke the spirit of the Sphinx to empower your spine and awaken your inner vitality. Let's begin.

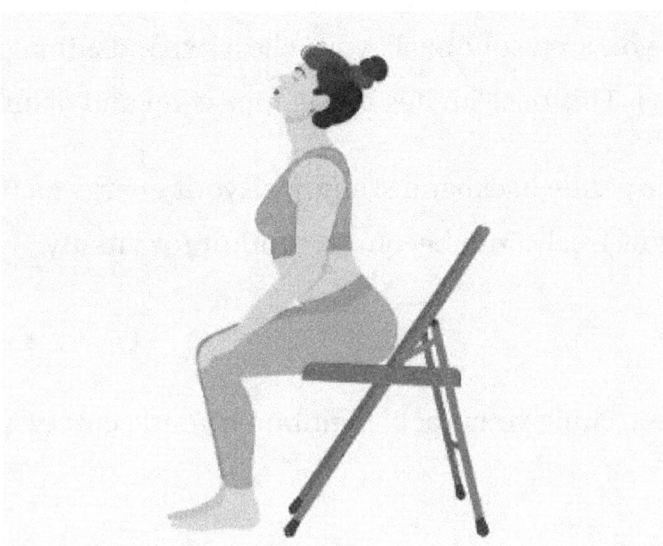

Actions

Finding Your Seat: Sit at the edge of a sturdy chair, feet planted firmly on the ground. Imagine your spine elongating, creating space between each vertebra. Feel the chair supporting you.

Hand Placement: Place your hands on your knees, palms facing down. This connection grounds your energy and prepares you for the gentle backbend.

Inhale and Slide: As you inhale, gently slide your hands toward your hips. Imagine a subtle arch in your lower back, like the graceful curve of the Sphinx. Feel your chest opening forward and up.

Neck and Gaze: Keep your neck long and relaxed. Gaze forward, allowing your chin to remain parallel to the ground. Imagine the Sphinx's unwavering gaze, observing the mysteries of life.

Hold the Pose: Hold this gentle backbend for a few breaths. Feel the stretch along your spine, from the base (tailbone) to the crown (top of the head). Breathe deeply, inviting space into your chest and heart center.

Benefits

Spinal Health: The Chair Sphinx Pose encourages a healthy curvature in your spine. It counteracts the effects of prolonged sitting, promoting flexibility and preventing stiffness.

Heart Opening: As you arch your back, your chest expands. Imagine your heart center blossoming like a lotus. This pose invites self-compassion and openness.

Energetic Flow: The gentle backbend stimulates your energy channels (nadis), allowing prana (life force) to flow freely. You become a conduit for vitality.

Common Mistakes

Overarching: While arching your back, maintain a gentle curve. Avoid excessive strain or discomfort.

Tension in the Neck: Keep your neck relaxed. The focus is on the spine, not the neck.

Variations

Chair Tree Pose (Seated Spinal Twist): Cross your right ankle over your left thigh. Place your right hand on the outside of your left knee and gently twist to the left. Feel the twist from your base (pelvis) to your crown (head). Breathe deeply and unwind any tension.

Chapter 9:

Conclusion: Embracing Chair Yoga

As we draw the curtains on this enlightening journey through the realms of Chair Yoga, it becomes clear that what we embarked on is far more than a series of physical exercises. It's a transformative path towards empowerment and independence, especially tailored for seniors who aspire to enhance their mobility, strength, and overall quality of life. Chair Yoga, with its gentle yet effective approach, opens a gateway to a more vibrant and autonomous existence, even as we age. Let us delve into how embracing Chair Yoga fully can be your ally in achieving a life filled with more joy, health, and independence.

Embracing Chair Yoga as a Path to Empowerment: Step-by-Step Actions

1. **Acknowledge the Journey**: Start by acknowledging the progress you've made. Each movement, breath, and session marks a step towards greater well-being. Celebrate these milestones, however small they may seem.

2. **Set Personal Goals**: Define what empowerment means to you. Is it walking without aid, gardening without pain, or playing with your grandchildren with ease? Tailor your Chair Yoga practice to meet these goals.

3. **Integrate Practice into Daily Life**: Make Chair Yoga a natural part of your daily routine. Allocate a specific time for practice, ensuring consistency. This consistency will reinforce your path to empowerment.

4. **Mindfulness and Meditation**: Incorporate mindfulness and meditation into your sessions. Chair Yoga isn't just about physical strength but also mental resilience. This holistic approach fosters independence.

Examples

Marilyn's Story: At 75, Marilyn found that Chair Yoga helped her regain the strength to perform her daily tasks without relying on her cane as much. Her goal was to walk her dog without fear of falling. Through dedicated practice, she achieved this, showcasing the empowering nature of Chair Yoga.

George's Transformation: After incorporating Chair Yoga into his daily routine, George noticed a significant reduction in his chronic back pain. This allowed him to resume his hobby of model ship building, which required hours of sitting, demonstrating the practice's potential to restore independence.

Resources and Continuing Your Practice: Online Classes for Ongoing Learning

In today's digital age, the journey of learning and growth never truly ends. Numerous resources are available for seniors to continue their Chair Yoga practice and further their journey towards empowerment.

Step-by-Step Actions

1. **Explore Online Platforms**: Websites like Yoga International and Gaia offer specialized Chair Yoga classes for seniors. Begin with beginner-friendly sessions, gradually progressing to more advanced classes.

2. **Join Virtual Communities**: Platforms such as Facebook and Meetup host groups for Chair Yoga enthusiasts. These communities offer support, share experiences, and provide motivation.

3. Stay Informed: Subscribe to newsletters or blogs dedicated to senior wellness and Chair Yoga. They can be a great source of inspiration and information on the latest practices and research.

Examples

Linda's Learning Curve: Linda, a 68-year-old retiree, found a new community through an online Chair Yoga class. This virtual platform not only allowed her to continue her practice from home but also connected her with peers across the globe, fostering a sense of belonging and shared purpose.

Tom's Tech-Savvy Approach: Despite initial reservations about using technology, Tom embraced online resources to enhance his Chair Yoga practice. He now uses apps to track his progress and participates in live-streamed classes, proving that learning and adapting can continue at any age.

Conclusion

Embracing Chair Yoga is not merely about adopting a fitness routine; it's about embarking on a journey towards a more empowered and independent self. Through dedicated practice, the right resources, and a community of support, seniors can transform their lives, proving that age is but a number. Let Chair Yoga be your companion on this path to a fuller, more vibrant life.